"In *The Aging Myth,* Joe Chang highlights how genes and gene expression are important for postponing aging and dispels the myth that we cannot slow the clock of aging. Chang explains that the most effective anti-aging strategies consist of healthy lifestyle changes and the consumption of essential micronutrients. *The Aging Myth* will provide all health-conscious individuals with guidelines for improving both life and youthspan."

LESTER PACKER, PH.D., Adjunct Professor, Department of Pharmacology and Pharmaceutical Sciences, School of Pharmacy,
University of Southern California Distinguished Professor, Chinese Academy of Sciences, Institute of Nutritional Sciences, Shanghai, China*

"*The Aging Myth* is written for anyone who is concerned with healthy aging. Aging is not merely a passive wear and tear process over time, but an active biological process regulated by several key genes. Joe Chang explains the pivotal role of gene expression in aging—at a level comprehensible to the general reader—without oversimplifying a complicated science. The book deserves to be read because it successfully explains a very complicated process to the layman, with minimal scientific jargon."

(CURTIS) MAKOTO KURO-O, M.D., PH.D., Associate Professor of Pathology, University of Texas Southwestern Medical Center*

"Dr. Chang presents a cutting-edge innovative approach—backed by proven genetic science—to the universal quest to stay young."

JACKIE SILVER, Founder and President, AgingBackwards.com

"Joe Chang and team are able to better understand the role of gene expression in skin aging. This research will lead to the next generation of skin care products that could address more than just the signs of aging."

ZOE DIANA DRAELOS, M.D., F.A.A.D., Dermatologist and Editor-in-Chief, *Journal of Cosmetic Dermatology**

"Nu Skin goes to extremes to foster innovation. ageLOC is proof that it is worth it, and it sends a very clear message that Nu Skin is the place to be."

BLAKE RONEY, Chairman of the Board, Nu Skin Enterprises

"Dr. Joseph Chang's extensive research and experience in the field of anti-aging have yielded unique, no-nonsense solutions to help people look and feel young throughout their lives. His innovative approach, backed by extensive genetic research, provides hope for a more youthful future for all who seek it."

DAVID BEARSS PH.D., Co-Director of the Center for Investigational Therapeutics, Huntsman Cancer Institute and Associate Professor, University of Utah*

"This book empowers consumers everywhere to make a choice about how they want to live the rest of their lives. Joe Chang expounds on his lifetime goal of finding a way to live better longer and gives you the tools to take action in your personal fight against aging."

KEN DYCHTWALD, PH.D. President and CEO of Age Wave and author of *Age Wave, Age Power* and *A New Purpose*

*Member of Nu Skin Advisory Board (see pp. 165–174)

THE
AGING
MYTH

THE AGING MYTH

UNLOCKING THE MYSTERIES OF
LOOKING AND FEELING YOUNG

JOSEPH CHANG, PH.D.

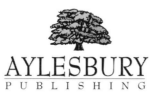

AYLESBURY
PUBLISHING

To Ping, who has kept me young all along the way.

TABLE OF CONTENTS

*"Wish not so much to live long,
as to live well."*

BENJAMIN FRANKLIN

WE ALL AGE, BUT DO WE HAVE TO STUMBLE BLINDLY DOWN the years, accepting whatever comes with it? Not if I can help it. For centuries, people have wanted to know how and why we age and what, if anything, can be done about it. Throughout the years, the never-ending quest for youth has brought us many silly and down-right ridiculous lotions, potions, and ideas. From store shelves to YouTube instructional videos we have seen some bizarre ideas about anti-aging. However, in the past few decades, some unprecedented and remarkable scientific research has unlocked new information about aging, leading to crucial anti-aging breakthroughs.

These research breakthroughs related to the sources of aging and the explanation of the science behind them are contained in the book you now hold in your hands.

You've heard it said that knowledge is power. Plato said, "The measure of a man is what he does with power." After reading this book you'll be "in the know" about the causes of aging and have in your arsenal powerful knowledge you can use to improve your odds in the battle against aging.

You will have the power to improve the appearance of many signs of aging such as crow's feet, laugh lines, and wrinkles. You will better understand your body and what it needs to retain its youthful vitality on the inside as well, including dodging that midday energy crash. You'll do it noninvasively, without needles, knives, lasers, or potentially harmful stimulants, which often come with a cost, including potentially negative side effects.

In this book you'll meet many people who already have achieved remarkable benefits without resorting to drastic methods of self-preservation. Their stories and photos will make you wonder what in the world they are doing to look and feel so great. So just keep reading and you'll find out what our amazing discovery is, where it came from, and how you can use it.

Several years ago, I came to a crossroads in my career. After years in medical research developing pharmaceuticals that had a significant positive impact on a number of major illnesses and serious aging related conditions, I decided fundamentally to switch careers. Many of my colleagues, friends, and family members naturally wondered why I would do an about-face after having spent most of my life discovering treatments for diseases. In other words, was I crazy to give up a career that was helping so many people who were suffering from life-threatening maladies?

The answer to that question was simple. I wasn't crazy; I simply wanted a change from treating disease, which is limited to those

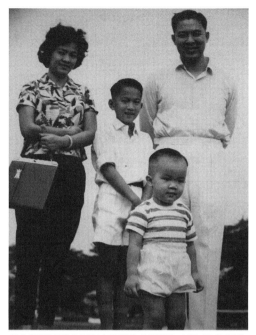

JOE (CENTER) WITH MOTHER, FATHER, AND BROTHER.

who *already* have issues, to helping people *before* the issues arise. Let me give you some background.

When I was very young I had a keen interest in science. My mother, a primary school teacher, and my father, a tin miner, were adamant that my brother, sister, and I go to college. They worked very hard to see that we did.

After my intense years of schooling and training, I became a research executive with large pharmaceutical companies, including Wyeth-Ayerst Research and Rhone Poulenc Rorer. Later, I started a biotech company in Boston called Binary Therapeutics, Inc. Despite these successes, I felt I had a higher mission. I was designing drugs that were targeted to treating specific serious health disorders which, don't get me wrong, is a great thing; *but* my past experiences drove me to want to do something that could actually be beneficial to everyone, with or without acute health issues. Treating critical health issues after the fact is like trying to round up the horses after they have bolted from the barn. My focus became more and more clear—to keep the horses in the barn. In other words, I wanted to keep people healthy so ideally they would never even *need* those drugs!

I sold Binary Therapeutics and, with a colleague named Michael Chang (no relation), started Pharmanex. Michael is a medicinal chemist by training, and, paired with me and my biological training, we made a perfect fit. Our combined expertise allowed us to bring a fresh perspective to the supplement industry, and we began developing scientifically proven dietary supplements out of pure and natural products that would build a body's natural health defenses at the cellular level. The company offered superior nutritional products to maintain and protect cells, tissues, and organs in the body and to promote healthy aging.

The difference between Pharmanex and the many other dietary supplement companies out there was having science as our central tenet. In our opinion, with few exceptions, the dietary supplement industry was fraught with problems and in need of serious scientific rigor and quality control. We were determined to make a difference with our approach. All of our research and development was conducted employing strict pharmaceutical standards.

By 1998, we were into the third year of production, and, with our products in thousands of stores, our research was gaining industry-wide attention and offers for acquisition were appearing. Three offers, including two from pharmaceutical giants, had appeal to us. Our dilemma was this: we needed the money and backing of a larger company to advance our research and gain the ability to bring the world's best natural supplements to a global market, but if we chose the wrong company, would we be able to maintain our integrity and our science-based identity?

Even though we had already achieved significant sales, this was literally just a drop in the bucket compared to the sales of the giant pharmaceutical companies. Since Pharmanex products carry the most potent and effective doses of the finest, most effective ingredients and are more expensive to develop, how long would the mother company support our commitment to scientific excellence?

We were spending every available resource (time and money) developing the most effective natural supplements. We had already invested our hearts and reputations into our formulas and we wanted to find a partner that would appreciate what we had and build on it, not tear it down. I would rather have failed with quality products, than have succeeded with what I would call "junk."

The third company that approached us was Nu Skin Enterprises, a global company that was then operating in 26 markets throughout the Americas, Asia, and Europe, with an international sales force of over 500,000 independent distributors. Frankly, because I didn't know anything about this company, or the direct selling industry in general, I was skeptical.

The more I learned, the more the right choice for us became obvious. Nu Skin had already spent many years and invested millions of dollars into developing a superior line of skin and beauty products that were scientifically researched and produced using the highest quality standards, and the company already recognized that real beauty is addressed from the inside *and* the outside. I was extremely impressed. They were kindred spirits. Michael and I felt the two companies' mutual desire to adhere to the highest standards of product quality made a perfect fit. By combining our expertise in nutrition with Nu Skin Enterprises' already robust skin care line, we had the potential to redefine the anti-aging industry. By bringing beauty and health to the outside and inside, we could truly change lives.

We knew that as one company, living and breathing the same credo, we could do great things and, most importantly, we didn't have to sacrifice quality for profit. Together, we could create a company that makes a difference. With an international selling engine (today including over 750,000 independent distributors) and our one-two punch of quality products, we could go global overnight.

This was the right direction, and our science would continue to advance. Together, we would improve lives and help people! Certainly a new anti-aging breakthrough, such as the one revealed in this book, could not have been created without this tradition and pursuit of scientific excellence.

With the blessing and financial backing of a company willing to partner with us in scientific health research, we were able to go on to the next big step. By joining with what is now a staff of more than 75 dedicated scientists and collaborating with multiple scientific institutions around the world, the Nu Skin Enterprises research and development engine is now consistently producing formulas and products that enable us to set new industry standards in anti-aging.

So, this is what I am doing with the second half of my career: doing my best to keep the horses from running amok, reining in the negative effects of aging, and dedicating my life to helping all people who are willing to take control of their own present and future health and well-being. I have not only chosen to surround myself with an entire culture focused on prevention and healthy living, but am helping people achieve the bodies and lifestyles where the ravages of aging are not invited!

For the last decade, we have continually been developing fundamental breakthrough formulas and tools that we can deliver to consumers. We're proud that we have this tradition of innovation. Now, with this book, I am going to introduce you to the next and most significant breakthrough, which will forever alter the anti-aging landscape.

OUR BREAKTHROUGH SCIENCE

Through our recent collaborations with some of the best anti-aging researchers in the world, we have learned to go to the genetic level and have contributed innovative and unique knowledge to the body of anti-aging science.

In the pages that follow, I will introduce you to our work and explain our philosophy, our research, and the amazing way we have changed people's lives.

Specifically, I will explain how we have identified clusters of genes in the body and skin that we believe directly relate to aging. By understanding which sets of genes are the most important in relation to aging, we can remind them to function as they once did in youth. Just like your computer. Over time, when your computer no longer functions like it did when it was new—when it becomes corrupt and freezes up—what do you do? You go for a hard reset, right? That's what we're going to do with these sets of genes.

Reset them.

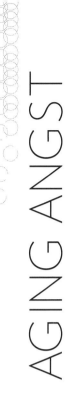

1

AGING ANGST

*"Age to me means nothing. I can't get old;
I'm working. As long as you're working,
you stay young. When I'm in front of an audience,
all that love and vitality sweeps over me
and I forget my age."*

GEORGE BURNS

I WAS WATCHING TELEVISION THE OTHER EVENING AND, during a one-hour program, saw three 60-second commercials touting anti-aging products. The focus on anti-aging is a giant wave sweeping the world. This is a huge trend—not a fad. Anti-aging research is here to stay and is coming of age (so to speak). Products and services that address aging are increasing globally— everything from cosmetics, to food, to supplements.

This global trend goes way beyond the desire to look younger. According to a report by the U.S. Census Bureau and the National

Institutes of Health, currently a half-billion people are over 65 years old, and that number is quickly climbing to a billion in this century. By 2040 there will be an estimated 1.3 billion people over the age of 65, representing 14% of the world population. Within 10 years, for the first time in human history, the number of people in the world aged 65 years and older will exceed that of children under the age of 5. In many countries, people age 80 and older are the fastest growing portion of the population. Between 2008 and 2040, that segment of the population is projected to increase 233%, compared with 160% for those age 65 and older and 33% for the total world population.

Why do I tell you all of this? Just ask anyone and they will tell you that if living longer is in the cards, they want to live those extra years to the fullest, not just survive them. With constant advances in technology, we have become accustomed to quality living with new innovations creating solutions to nearly every problem we come across each day. We expect, and frankly we demand, this same type of effort in what matters most to us . . . our *life*!

SOME OF US AGE BETTER THAN OTHERS. WHY?

It's happening to each of us. From the day we emerge into this world, we start to age. However, some of us age better than others. Why do some live up to a healthy and youthful 100 years, while others can barely get out of bed at age 65?

Most of us have had the experience of going to a class reunion—the homecoming queen looks like she hasn't aged a day, but the athletic cheerleader is wrinkled and arthritic. The football captain who sat sleeping in the back of the room in English 101 looks like he is 101, while the teacher who taught the class seems to be aging backwards.

What is going on? What is the difference? Why do some people look so much younger than other people their age? For those who didn't age gracefully, could they have done anything differently? And then we ask ourselves, how am I doing?

MIRROR, MIRROR . . . WHERE IS MY YOUTH?

So we take a good look in the mirror. Instead of the usual glance as we head out the door, we stop and stare at that image looking back at us, and, after a few introspective moments, we realize we are *aging*! For years we've gone along under the delusion that we look perpetually 21 because we think and feel 21. Life has rushed by since then.

To some people, it's a real shock to discover wrinkles, sagging jowls, and puffy eyes. What's more, they want to know why they feel as tired as they are starting to look.

A friend of mine is an artist. It's her habit to sketch random people while in a waiting room, church, or at the bus stop. One day she drew a beautiful septuagenarian who had amazingly hypnotic eyes, an exotic nose, marvelous full lips and naturally curly black hair. She also had deep laugh lines around her eyes and other assorted wrinkles and creases that the artist thought gave her an interesting character. The artist could see the woman in a beautiful painting as a gypsy, draped in colorful scarves and brilliant dangling jewelry. However, when she showed the sketch to her subject for approval to use it in a painting, it was obvious that the woman wasn't seeing either "exoticness" or "character." She literally shrieked, "That doesn't look like me! I don't look like that!" She then reached over, tore the drawing from the book, stuffed it in her pocket, and stalked away. (My artist friend assures me that the drawing was not only accurate, but even flattering.)

I wonder if that woman examined herself in the mirror that evening. What, if any, illusions were altered? You see, although we all see ourselves in our mind's eye at a certain age, eventually the mirror reflects the truth right back in our face. We can't hide anymore. The response in that moment of shock is almost always the same. "This is really happening. I need to do something about this!"

I honestly think people fear looking and feeling older. But what can be done? It all seems so inevitable and entirely overwhelming. But I'm here to tell you that my life's work in drug discovery and supplement research gives me a better perspective of maximizing the ability to develop anti-aging solutions. Because you picked up this book, you no longer need to have "aging angst." No doubt the entire civilized world is concerned about aging. Why? Because people are living longer and hoping to live it *alive!*

I don't blame them. The reality of aging hits me even harder because I am a scientist and I know that we can do something about it. I am also aging, and, being in my 50s, I certainly want to hold onto my own health and youth. The key desire that so many aging people share is to know what they can do to empower themselves to age gracefully.

CAN WE DIE HEALTHY?

I say in my presentations around the world: "Can we die healthy?" It makes sense that our goal should be to go out of life dancing on the

OUTRAGEOUS AGING CLAIMS

Through the centuries there have been extremely wild claims involving extreme longevity. Sumerian genealogies claim that three kings reigned 72,000 years each. Biblical accounts of longevity range from Methuselah at 969 years to Job at 210 to Joshua at 110. The Torah makes similar claims and so do Arabic cultures. In Chinese legend, Peng Zu was believed to have lived for 800 years. Alchemy, in this case (the idea that humans can transform their own substance into something else, including immortal ingredients) was popular as late as the fourteenth-century when alchemist Nicolas Flamel purported to produce the "Elixir of Life," which he drank to ensure his own immortality. If it worked, he is about 680 years old today.

See References in Appendix

LIVING LONG ENOUGH TO WORRY ABOUT AGING

According to a report by the United Nations in 2009, in the richer countries around the world, life expectancy lengthens five hours or more every day. With longer and, in many cases, more productive lives, people are actually living long enough to worry about aging.

There was a time when infection, malnutrition, complications of childbirth, food poisoning, and dangerous living conditions dictated a short lifespan for people worldwide. Over the course of the past century antibiotics, sanitation, and medical care have dramatically reduced death rates in the early and middle years of life, allowing people to live long enough to age. In fact, when I studied at Johns Hopkins I was guided to a deep appreciation of the importance of preventative medicine by the powerful influence of the dean of the school, Donald Henderson, who was responsible for the eradication of small pox—the scourge of humankind for centuries. Dr. Henderson's work and other experiences became powerful influences on my life, driving me to search for answers to maintaining good health throughout life, no matter how long that life may be.

Ironically, today the dominant cause of death in developed countries is the **aging process itself and the associated maladies that come with it.**

Kirkwood, Thomas (September 2010). "Why Can't We Live Forever." *Scientific American*, pp. 42–49.
http://un.org/ageing/popageing.html

LIVING TO 150. WANNA BET?

Two scientists feel strongly enough about this 150-year question to put their money where their mouths are. Steve Austad of the University of Idaho and Jay Olshansky of the University of Illinois placed a bet on whether anyone born in the year 2000 would still be around in 2150. In other words, will someone alive today live to be 150? Keep in mind that the oldest living person to date was Jeanne Calmant who was born February 21, 1875, and died August 4, 1997, at the age of 122 years and 164 days.

Olshansky and Austad drew up a contract, and each put $150 in a bank account. The winner's heirs will get the cash. With interest over 150 years, the payoff will come to about $500 million. Both men believe that for a person to make it to 150, scientists will have to come up with some way to slow aging. The question is—can they do it in time?

Olshansky: "No way. Even if we developed a technology 10 to 20 years from now, I can't imagine we could slow aging enough to add another 30 years to the human life span. Besides, you'd have to find the right person, someone who will already live to be a super centenarian. What are the chances you'll find one? This is a no-brainer. My relatives will be wealthy."

Austad: "Yes way. Even if the technology is not available for 50 years, there'll still be a bunch of 50-year-olds whose aging we can slow down. Now, more and more people are living to 100. And the more 100-year-olds you have, the more will live to 110. The more that live to 110, the more that will live to 120. For this bet, only one person has to live to 150. That's only about 20 percent more than 122. I think it's a slam dunk."

The result of the bet will be determined January 1, 2150.

"How Long Can People Live?" Karen Hopkin

final day, not just living out our final days on a couch or in a bed. Well we can, but first, a bit more background on what some scientists in the field are discussing on the topic of aging.

A recent special report in the September 2010 issue of *Scientific American* magazine poses my question this way: "Why can't we live forever?" The average lifespan of humans continues to lengthen, and some scientists have begun to ponder just how long this trend will last.

For centuries, scientists believed that human aging was fixed— a process programmed into our biology that resulted in a built-in time of death. But today, because of the latest scientific advances, scientists are beginning to revise their lifespan estimates. Better sanitation, food supply, medical care, and vaccinations have all contributed to longevity. In 1900, the average life expectancy was 45, and in 1950 it was 65. In the 1990s, it rose to 75. We now know that all things being equal, people may be able to live to 150. But let's stay focused on the objective. It is not necessarily about the *amount* of years added to a human life, but the *quality* of those years. Our objective is not to live forever, but to truly die *healthy*.

THE QUEST FOR IMMORTALITY

Let me give you an example of what I mean. The *age-old* (pardon the pun) quest that has been a fantasy of human beings and the basis of stories and legends for centuries is the quest for immortality. But we must be careful what we ask for.

There is a story in Greek mythology that illustrates the folly of mortal beings wishing to live indefinitely. Tithonus, a handsome mortal man, fell in love with Eos, the immortal goddess of the dawn. Eos realized that her beloved Tithonus was destined to age and die. She begged Zeus to grant her lover immortal life.

In a classic devil's bargain, he granted Eos's wish—literally. He made Tithonus immortal but did not grant him eternal youth.

As Tithonus aged, he became increasingly debilitated and demented, eventually driving Eos to distraction with his constant babbling. In despair, Eos turned Tithonus into a grasshopper. (In Greek mythology, the grasshopper is immortal, explaining why grasshoppers chirp ceaselessly like demented old men.)

Is it really this "delusion" of immortality we're seeking? I think not. The quest for youth has been going on for centuries, from the sixteenth-century explorer Ponce de Leon spending much of his life and fortune searching for immortality to Cleopatra bathing in goat milk because she believed that it helped her turn back the clock, the list goes on and on. But let me restate what I mentioned earlier. **The point is to live better, longer. What we want to focus on is not lifespan, but what I call youthspan. This is the mission that has become my life's work.**

KEEP YOUR AGE A MYSTERY

So let's go back to the question we asked earlier in this chapter: why do some people look younger and some people look older than their actual age? Well my team has been researching this exact question for years.

Did you know that across the globe people feel that the biggest anti-aging question in their mind is not "Why do we get wrinkles?"

or "How do our bodies lose the grip on gravity's pull?" but rather "Why do some people look younger than their real age?" Just to prove the point, our marketing team scoured the globe to find these people. Everyone knows someone who looks young for their age, and we asked people to submit photos from all over the world to demonstrate this. Turn to the Appendix, page 193, to see some of the photos we collected, and see if you can guess their age gaps. The answers are on page 202.

Aren't those photos remarkable? They simply confirm the notion that people vary in how they age over time.

Most often, looking young is attributed to people having good genes, but if it's all in the genes, then aging is inevitable and you can't do anything to change it. That answer has never been acceptable to me, so our team has delved deeply into the molecular mechanisms of aging and has learned something *can* be done about aging at the genetic level. It's not about changing the genes, *it's about influencing gene expression.*

IT *IS* IN THE GENES, JUST NOT THE WAY YOU'VE THOUGHT

When someone looks pretty, handsome, or younger than their age, your grandmother or mother would shrug and say, "Oh, she just has good genes." And they are partly right, everyone has good genes, but the key is how your genes are being expressed. Your genes are *your* genes and they are fixed. They can't be altered.

But when it comes to looking younger than your age, what scientists have discovered is that it's not about altering the genes, but about something called *youthful gene expression.*

GENE EXPRESSION

What exactly *is* gene expression? It is one of the more fascinating components of our body functioning, subtle and exciting in its effect. It is also a very important part of our healthy anti-aging science and so key that I devote all of Chapter 2 to explaining to you its amazing properties. But most simply, gene expression is how our genes talk to our cells. Gene expression tells a cell what it is going to be.

A child's *youthful gene expression* tells his or her skin cells to be young, healthy, and fully active. When you see adults looking younger than their age, their genes are continuing to express themselves as if they were young. Their genes are still communicating like youthful genes and as a result, their body remains young. They often have smooth, elastic skin and a great complexion, which are reflective of youthfulness.

Isn't it amazing? Our mothers and grandmothers almost had it right. What they should have said is, "She has good gene expression." They were just leaving out one critical distinction—expression. You see, aging is *not* in the genes; aging is *in* the gene expression.

Mom (and Grandma) made that statement because that is the knowledge they had about aging and genes at that time. They firmly believed it was simply a matter of having good genes and nothing could be done about it.

As a scientist this is puzzling to me. People readily accept that we can "do something" to improve all kinds of human conditions, from major diseases like smallpox or cancer to everyday complaints like sore throats, indigestion, and hangnails. However, amazingly, they don't believe we can truly impact aging.

So the good news is this: years of research have generated scientific discoveries about the aging process, and I can unequivocally say that we know more about, and can target, not only the signs and symptoms of aging, **but also the sources of aging that were previously well-hidden in the genes.**

Before, you envied those people who were "blessed" with good genes and assumed if your body was not aging gracefully, you just didn't have the genes for it. The big news for you is that the discoveries we have made reveal that you *do* have "good" genes. You just need to know how to keep *your* genes expressing themselves in a more youthful pattern!

KEEP THEM GUESSING

Wouldn't it be marvelous if we could help aging skin look more like young skin? To promote health and vitality in hearts, muscles, and brains? To help them function more like they did in younger days? Well, here's the good news. We can.

Recently, genetic research has revealed the possibility of influencing aging-related gene expression and ultimately the functional pathways that directly relate to aging. By taking advantage of these discoveries, you can take charge of your own aging and will keep everyone guessing your age for years to come.

YOUTHFUL SKIN REFLECTS HEALTH

Medical science has made fantastic advancements in the realm of disease control, but has only just begun to adequately deal with longevity in terms of the insidious damage done to our bodies by rampant pollution, free radicals, and the slow poison of processed food, not to mention alcohol and tobacco. While we are living longer, our bodies, and especially our skin, are taking a beating.

One of the reasons I initially partnered with Nu Skin was because of their commitment to research and development, including their dedication to anti-aging research and discovery. The majority of our attention initially was on the causes of aging in the skin.

Why did we choose to focus first on the skin? Because our skin is the largest organ that we can see, touch, and feel, making it easier to study. Our skin literally reflects many aspects of our health. It can mirror back to us where we are in terms of youthful health and vitality. Youthful skin looks healthy. It is thick, more elastic, and radiant. It rebounds more quickly from abrasions, cuts, and contusions. It has fewer discolorations. By using skin as a research model, we have made wonderful breakthroughs in all aspects of anti-aging, inside *and* out.

In the next several chapters, we will break down in detail the discoveries we have made and how they can impact you and provide *you* with your very own answers to *your* quest for youthfulness and vitality.

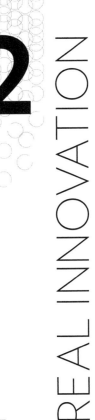

"An ounce of prevention is worth a pound of cure."
BENJAMIN FRANKLIN

I AM ONE WHO BELIEVES IN THE OLD ADAGE, "AN OUNCE OF prevention is worth a pound of cure." That is why the most important science being conducted today is in prevention and anti-aging.

Let me take you back a few years in my life. As I mentioned in the introduction to this book, I spent the first part of my career in drug discovery. Now, I focus on the other side of that coin: prevention. I firmly believe that prevention *is* the answer to health and to aging!

A real epiphany came to me when my father and my wife's mother died. Both dear older people lived well into their 70s. Both were beloved, honored people who mattered deeply in our lives and we were, naturally, saddened beyond expression at their passing. What really stuck with me, however, was *how* they died. This left a lasting impact on how I think about aging.

My father suffered for a long time before he finally passed. He had a chronic deterioration of his health that took him down a long and painful journey until he finally passed away. My mother-in-law, on the other hand, lived a healthier, vigorous, happy lifestyle right up to the very moment when she quietly and peacefully slipped away in my wife's arms.

I was deeply troubled as to why my dad's body deteriorated like it did, causing him so much pain and disability. What were the factors that contributed to my mother-in-law's stronger, more vital constitution? In other words, why did she seem to age so much more gracefully than did he? Why did she die healthy?

It was then that I fully recognized that there must be a way to help people die healthy so that while they are alive, they are truly living.

Well I believe we found it. You no longer need to feel ambivalent or hopeless about not looking and feeling more youthful and vigorous far into your later years.

In this chapter, I will walk you through a whole new approach to anti-aging research called ageLOC. I will explain the discovery, the history, and the cutting-edge science behind ageLOC so that you will be able to appreciate how significant and life-changing I believe ageLOC will become.

It's also important to understand that ageLOC is not just an intriguing name to put on a new R&D effort. ageLOC is a fundamental approach to identify and target the sources of aging, not just to treat the signs and symptoms.

ageLOC also represents the remarkably innovative science and technology platform by which we are able to identify, target, and reset the sources of aging. So, from this point forward, when you

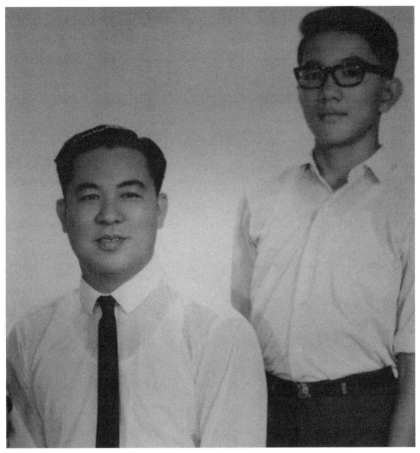

JOE (RIGHT) AND HIS FATHER.

hear me mention the term ageLOC, I am speaking of our anti-aging research.

ageLOC incorporates the latest thinking in the field of anti-aging genetic research and I believe it *is* a better way. Our comprehensive approach targets the sources of aging, not just its effects, or signs, by understanding the expression of multiple genes, rather than one single gene.

SEEKING INNOVATION

Let's begin with a little history. In the introduction, I told you that Dr. Michael Chang and I started a company called Pharmanex. In fact, we left lucrative positions with large pharmaceutical companies to create our own nutritional supplement company. We wanted to incorporate the best science that could be applied to our product development. In other words, it was time to kick out the charlatans and snake-oil salesmen and bring in the scientists, if the industry was ever going to gain credibility.

I believed in the effectiveness of natural products. In fact, I grew up with ancient and modern Chinese natural medicine as a part of my life. Some natural products have miraculous, even mysterious, healing properties. What I took issue with was the industry's indifference to quality ingredients and quality manufacturing. These natural products still need to be understood scientifically and formulated under strict manufacturing guidelines instead of being marketed and formulated using a willy-nilly approach.

TRADITIONAL WISDOM AND SCIENCE TOGETHER

My mission with Pharmanex was to advance the dietary supplement field as far from superstition and ignorance as was humanly possible by melding traditional wisdom with modern science. To me, it was only through science that I could help people appreciate the value of natural ingredients. My goal was to extract what was good in such ingredients and eliminate what was bad. That was my vision then; it is my vision now.

When we found that the company Nu Skin lived by a similar credo, "All of the good. None of the bad," we knew that Pharmanex and Nu Skin were a perfect fit, that we were coming together at the right time for the right purpose. Our combined strengths put us in perfect launch position to rocket ahead in the anti-aging arena.

TARGETING THE SOURCES OF AGING

Joining Nu Skin was so exciting for us. With their backing, we were able to put our energies immediately into better understanding the underlying causes of aging. We knew it was more than skin deep and even suspected that it probably went all the way to the genetic level, but there were so many variables, including the obvious one: we didn't even know at that time how many genes there were in a single cell, let alone understand which of these genes had an impact on aging. The technology simply didn't exist.

A GREAT BREAKTHROUGH

In 2003, after 13 years of coordinated effort between the U.S. Department of Energy and the National Institutes of Health, the Human Genome Project was completed. This offered us key tools and insights to better understand how the body ages at the gene expression level and enabled us to approach anti-aging in an entirely revolutionary way.

http://www.ornl.gov/sci/techresources/Human_Genome/home.shtml

MAPPING THE HUMAN GENOME

In 2003, scientists were finally able to map the human genome. This discovery gave us the foundation to deeply understand how the body ages and enabled us to approach anti-aging in an entirely revolutionary way.

So what in the world does mapping the human genome mean? And what is a genome anyway? Let me see if I can explain this simply.

There are more than six billion people on our planet, each of them a massive collection of about 100 trillion cells. How do these cells know what to do? What tells them to work together to keep your heart pumping, brain thinking, bones growing, or even to keep your skin elastic and smooth?

All of our genetic material is stored within our DNA. DNA (deoxyribonucleic acid) carries the instructions needed to build and maintain the many different types of cells that make you *you*. It is no wonder that DNA is known as the blueprint of life.

For storage purposes, our DNA is wound up into structures called chromosomes. Unwinding the DNA reveals all of our individual genes. The genome is simply a map of all the individual genes along that unwound DNA strand.

So, picture your "genome" as an "instruction manual" located in every one of your cells. Consider the chromosomes to be different chapters or sections inside this instruction manual. There are 20,000-25,000 words within the instruction manual. Each word is a "gene."

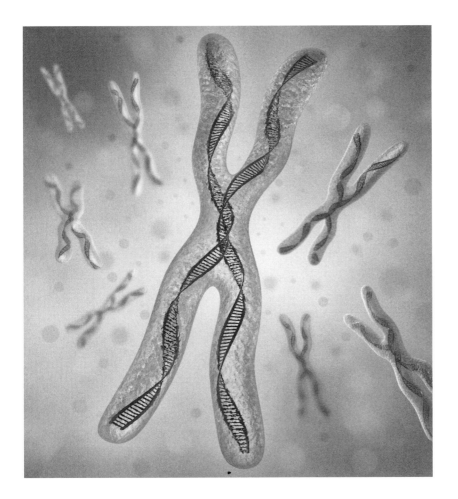

THE GENOME AND DNA

The genome, or genetic code, comprising 20,000 to 25,000 individual **genes**, is stored chemically within the cell as **DNA (deoxyribonucleic acid)**. This genome represents the full set of plans, or "blueprint," for building and running the cell. A DNA strand in a single cell is up to three meters long if stretched out all the way. In order to protect and organize these long DNA strands, they are wound up and packaged into coils called **chromosomes**. A full set of human DNA is stored as 46 chromosomes (23 chromosome pairs—one from the mother, the other from the father). **Amazingly, all humans share more than 99 percent of their genetic information. We are all much more alike on the genetic level than we realize. In essence, we do all have the same genes.**

http://www.ornl.gov/sci/techresources/Human_Genome/home.shtml

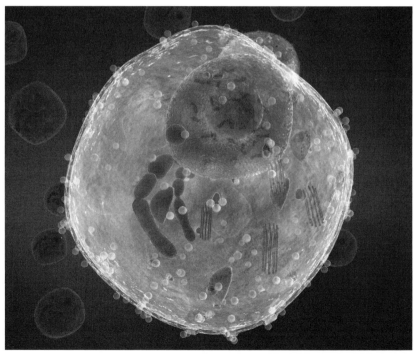

REPRESENTATION OF A CELL.

Now, obviously, you don't need each word in an entire manual to focus on a specific item. For example, you wouldn't look at instructions for changing a tire on your car if you were looking for how to change your oil.

While this instruction manual is located in every cell of the body, each cell only uses the part of the manual it needs. For example, a skin cell will only look at the specific words, or genes, which it needs to function.

So, each time a cell anywhere in your body needs something—say fuel, or a repair, or wants to divide—the genome manual opens up and gene instructions that relate to that particular cell send out chemical messages that the cell can understand.

As we researched this area in greater depth, it became very apparent that with age our genes don't change—*our* genes are *our* genes; the way that our genes are expressed or "communicate" changes with age. This is the area we began focusing on—gene expression, one of the ultimate sources of aging.

Now, understanding how genes function is one thing, but sorting through what had been thought to be hundreds of thousands of them to find "that one" you were looking for? Impossible. That is why the mapping of the human genome, perhaps the greatest scientific discovery of our generation, provided a critical puzzle piece to our genetic approach. The Human Genome Project identified all the genes in human DNA and stored the information in databases so all researchers everywhere can access it.

Scientists worldwide were ecstatic about the sequencing of the human genome along with the discovery that human DNA is comprised of approximately 20,000–25,000 genes, but it is still a daunting task to study aging at the genetic level. (Imagine the complexity of this venture. Even after this remarkable discovery, scientists still

UNDERSTANDING THE GENOME

The ageLOC approach allows us to understand the sequences of the Human Genome so we can decode their meanings in a way to help us study and understand the aging process. These sequences represent proteins, which express themselves as characteristics in every living organism. Now that we know which gene relates to a specific protein, we can balance or adjust that protein to achieve our desired results.

can't narrow down an exact number of genes, which is why we can only estimate the number of genes as being between 20,000–25,000.)

Isolating and studying each of the 20,000–25,000 genes to discover which are responsible for aging is like trying to find a needle in a haystack. There had to be a better way to narrow down our search. We knew we had to be able to target the *specific* genes that impact aging before we could help to influence them, so in essence the race was on to identify aging-related genes so that we could target aging at the source.

As important as it was to map the human genome, we still knew that we couldn't change genes, and that's why our focus has been, and continues to be, on gene expression.

We know, in fact, that our genes are not our destiny. Aging is *in* the genes, but it's not *all* about our genes. It's about how we *influence* our genes, or more accurately gene expression, that has the greatest impact on how we age.

GENE EXPRESSION: A DEFINITION

As we mentioned in Chapter 1, gene expression is how a cell communicates. Gene expression tells a cell what it is going to be. Aging

GENE EXPRESSION

The following paragraph represents a poorly written message. Though the paragraph below can be read and understood, it is not expressed well. Similarly, in aging, gene expression is muddled and the youthful message can be lost.

> There are four nucleotides that generally make up the genes within each one of our individual DNA, which are present, meaning they exist, within every cell in our body. These nucleotides are represented by four individual letters—a, c, g, and t. Genes are essentially found in each and every cell of each and every living thing, and they, meaning the genes, regulate an organism's function, meaning what it is supposed to do.

As you can see in the edits below, the genetic language, when properly expressed, makes perfect sense and the message is more clear.

> ~~There are~~ four nucleotides ~~that generally~~ make up the genes within ~~each one of~~ our ~~individual~~ DNA. ~~Which are present, meaning they exist, within every cell in our body.~~ These nucleotides are represented by four ~~individual~~ letters—a, c, g, and t. Genes are ~~essentially~~ found in each ~~and every~~ cell of ~~each and~~ every living thing and ~~they, meaning the genes,~~ regulate an organism's function. ~~Meaning what it is supposed to do.~~

The final message then reads:

> Four nucleotides make up the genes within our DNA. These nucleotides are represented by four letters—a, c, g, and t. Genes are found in each cell of every living thing and regulate an organism's function.

The ageLOC approach involves the study and understanding of how changes in gene expression contribute to the aging process. Gene expression, therefore, has a direct impact on cellular function. Our breakthrough is twofold: (1) our ability to identify the key genes whose expression changes with age *and* (2) our ability to reset their expression back to a more youthful profile.

happens when miscommunication happens in the cell.

Genes that were expressed at low levels during youth might increase in their expression as we age, while others decrease their level of expression. Gene expression does not categorically increase or categorically decrease as we age; each gene varies in its response—some up, some down, and some not at all.

We knew that the ability to measure aging at the gene expression level was important in how we address aging. We also knew that revolutionary breakthroughs are most often the result of experts from diverse disciplines coming together to develop solutions to far-reaching problems.

INNOVATION AND COLLABORATION: ENTER LIFEGEN

Isaac Newton once said, "If I have seen further, it is by standing on the shoulders of giants." This is exactly what we did. We know that great science is collaborative, that it doesn't evolve based on the research of a lone scientist or even a single company. As we narrowed our search in the genetic area, we determined there must be a great partner who shared our vision.

We sought out potential partners with expertise in genetics, gerontology, and bioinformatics. We met with a number of potential collaborators, but they all had limitations. Some were studying a single gene or a single tissue; many were using individual gene markers that only represented a small subset of the population. We wanted to partner with a group that shared our vision of a comprehensive approach to anti-aging.

As we continued our search, one company in particular intrigued me. LifeGen Technologies was co-founded by Dr. Richard Weindruch and Dr. Tomas A. Prolla, professors at the University of Wisconsin-Madison. Leaders in the fields of gerontology (aging), genetics, and nutrigenomics, they had been studying the aging process for many years. I was interested in their unique approach to studying aging. Together, they had more than 30 years of academic research, *and they truly lived their mission statement: "... to discover the genetic basis of the aging process with the goal of increasing the healthy life span of humans ..."*

The scientists at LifeGen are pioneers in nutrigenomics, which is the study of the effects of nutrients, phytochemicals, and antioxidants on gene expression. Another advantage was their ability to examine the expression of thousands of genes simultaneously using DNA microarray technology. (See Appendix for more information.)

So, as a team we recognized how well their expertise complemented our approach and expertise in the areas of aging research, including ingredient formulations. Many of LifeGen's key learnings on nutrigenomics were influenced by the research they were doing in the area of caloric restriction.

LESS CALORIES = LONGER LIFE

Benjamin Franklin said, "To lengthen thy life, lessen thy meals."

This statement by the quotable statesman was very perceptive. Did you know that if you reduce your caloric intake by 30% to 40% while still maintaining proper nutrition, you will probably live longer? Unless, of course, you get hit by a bus!

I know. You're probably saying, "Forget it. If I have to do that I don't want to live longer." Relax. I'm not advocating it. Depriving you of your glazed doughnut isn't our big anti-aging secret either. However, there is an important point to be made here, so bear with me.

Studies done on caloric restriction have been conducted for years. For example, two mice were raised in identical conditions with the exception that one was fed a regular calorie-nutritious diet, while the other was limited to a restricted caloric intake with nutritional supplementation. In nearly all cases, the mice with restricted intake of calories had visibly younger physical features. When autopsied after death, they also had clinically younger organs. (See Appendix for more information.)

CALORIC RESTRICTION

Researchers have been exploring the area of caloric restriction for years. Many people have heard the rumors that the lives of fruit flies, worms, mice, and even dogs have been extended through caloric restriction. Most of us say to ourselves, "Really? I am going to starve myself for the next 40 years so that I can live one extra year?" The real news is that caloric restriction combined with nutritional supplementation to replace lost nutrients has been shown to increase not just lifespan, but also healthspan. The idea of living healthier well into our years is a lot more tangible to most of us than just tacking on an extra year or two at the end of our lives.

So what exactly is caloric restriction, or CR? It is the reduction of calories by 30% to 40% over the lifespan; it is macronutrient restriction *without* micronutrient restriction. To date, CR is the only intervention consistently demonstrated in laboratory animals to increase both average and maximal lifespan.

MONKEYING AROUND

With such an obvious connection to aging, data compiled from laboratory caloric restriction models had to hold clues to finding the genes that are responsible for aging. I was intrigued that Dr. Weindruch and his colleagues at the University of Wisconsin-Madison had been doing long-term observations of rhesus monkeys on caloric restriction. Being primates, monkeys most resemble humans in genetic makeup, and they have a much longer lifespan than simpler mammals or organisms. Their most notable findings involved studying several pairs of monkeys over a 28-year period.

The monkeys that were allowed to eat a nutritious, healthy calorie diet aged visibly while the "dieting" monkeys had shinier coats, brighter eyes and more vigor. After clinical evaluation, their organs were considerably "younger" than the control group.

The key takeaway here is that the control monkeys were what we would consider a model for healthy aging. They were kept safe, they were not obese, they were eating a healthy diet, they didn't have detrimental environmental factors (like smoke and pollution), and yet they still aged visibly more than the restricted-calorie monkeys. This leads to the obvious conclusion that caloric restriction has a definite positive impact on the aging process.

Dr. Weindruch and his colleagues received worldwide acclaim for their findings. In fact, their findings were so groundbreaking that they are published in the most prestigious scientific journals in the world, such as *Science* and *Nature*.

TWENTY-EIGHT YEARS of detailed research? Most researchers in the anti-aging field were basing their conclusions on what they called "compelling" data using accelerated experiments on worms and flies lasting just days or weeks at best.

As we contemplated our holistic approach to anti-aging, we realized that with their long-term research, LifeGen would be a great partner that could infuse our own research and help us take our anti-aging approach to the next level.

RESEARCH PARTNERSHIP

On September 5, 2009, Nu Skin formed a research partnership with LifeGen Technologies. Nu Skin collaborates with LifeGen in an exclusive agreement by leveraging LifeGen's proprietary methods regarding gene expression profiling and pathways affected by aging. The mission of LifeGen Technologies is to "discover the genetic basis of the aging process with the goal of increasing the healthy life span of humans and animals." LifeGen's pioneering research resulted in several patents and patents pending, and ongoing research undertaken in collaboration with Nu Skin is expected to yield further important intellectual property. LifeGen's patent for the use of "gene expression profiling" as a method to measure the progression of the aging process at the molecular level in individual organs in mice is already a key component of the partnership.

LifeGen was co-founded in November 2000 by Richard Weindruch, Ph.D., and Tomas Prolla, Ph.D., professors at the University of Wisconsin-Madison and leaders in the fields of gerontology and genetics.

With the addition of Drs. Weindruch and Prolla, Nu Skin has refocused the efforts of its research collaborators in the direction of anti-aging. To facilitate this they formed the Nu Skin Anti-Aging Scientific Advisory Board.

CONNECTING THE DOTS

With the insights discovered in parallel with LifeGen's caloric restriction research, it became apparent, there does exist a model for healthy aging. This fed the pipeline of rigorous, long-term studies done by Dr. Weindruch and LifeGen on the underlying genetic understanding of aging. They continued their efforts to identify extremely useful genetic expression information. They observed unique gene expression patterns at different stages of the aging process. Basically they were able to demonstrate that gene expression patterns change with age and were able to document and capture those gene expression changes. In order to account for the effects of genetic diversity in the aging process, they incorporated seven genetically diverse strains of mice in all of these studies. From this research there were two key insights. **First,** they developed a way to *measure aging at the genetic level.* **Second,** they were able to narrow in on and confirm that *there were, indeed, multiple genes related to aging regardless of genetic diversity.* This research confirmed that we were on the right track in our quest and gave us the tools to make a breakthrough in anti-aging product development.

In summary, caloric restriction informed our hypothesis that gene *expression* in *multiple* genes is the key factor in aging. It showed us from another perspective that gene expression patterns differ dramatically depending on how you age and allowed us to compare aging profiles. When you age poorly, you will have a certain gene expression profile, but when you are in a healthy aging state, you will have a different gene expression profile. Our remarkable ability to compare and contrast these profiles provides us yet another tool to evaluate and identify specific ingredients that can actually reset the gene expression profile of these multiple genes to a more youthful state. Clearly our proprietary process to identify and blend specific ingredients together is a key advantage that allows us to use ageLOC science in an unprecedented anti-aging approach.

IT TAKES A VILLAGE

Another component of ageLOC that sets us apart from others in the anti-aging field is our belief, based on our research, that aging is due to the influence of gene expression in clusters of genes rather than changes in the expression of a single gene.

THE DATABANK

LifeGen, has aggregated a significant genetic database on the aging process. This database, which took nearly 30 years to develop, is a great tool which serves as an additional guide to our innovative anti-aging approach.

Having access to the detail and depth of research in the LifeGen database makes our work entirely unique in the anti-aging industry. I am unaware of any other resource that can examine the genetic expression profile of normal aging, caloric restriction, and the impact of natural products on these profiles. The database provides a reference that allows us to interpret our findings. If we see changes in gene expression in response to an ingredient, those changes are meaningless unless we have something to compare, e.g., youthful gene expression, CR gene expression, old gene expression. This reference data allows us to determine how much (or how little) an ingredient or a blend of ingredients modulates gene expression toward a more youthful pattern.

In my travels, I have opportunities to meet with and study the research of other lab teams around the world. I am frequently but silently stunned to see that many researchers in the anti-aging industry are still focusing on explaining aging via a single gene theory. Because of our excellent research partnerships with genetics experts worldwide, as well as our more holistic focus, we believe we are *years* ahead of others in the field of anti-aging in understanding that **there is no one single aging gene; we believe it's always about multiple genes when explaining aging.**

We know that you can't change your genes, but you can change your gene expression. This is key. But we *also* know that it is the gene expression of a multitude of genes, not a single gene, that influences how quickly or slowly we age. A lot of companies have been missing that link, focusing on a single gene or on a single gene characteristic.

YOUTH GENE CLUSTERS

Applying the findings that there are multiple genes involved in the aging process, as well as using our ability to measure their gene expression, our science team began to identify functional groups of genes associated with youthfulness. **We call these groups of genes *Youth Gene Clusters*.** Knowing about these gene clusters has given us a significant advantage over our competitors. While other anti-aging researchers must rummage through the entire Human Genome (what we refer to here as *the entire instruction manual*) hoping to find the clues they are looking for, our research has enabled us to hone in accurately and quickly on Youth Gene Clusters that we believe include the most important aging-related genes.

Even more exciting is that we can use our advantage to target those aging-related changes in gene expression with nutritional ingredients and finally reset the gene expression so that you can both look and feel better.

We have further learned, in contrast to other researchers who are still studying single-gene theory in the anti-aging field, that no matter how well you do it, you cannot influence the expression of only one gene and expect to impact the aging process.

We firmly believe it is imperative to target Youth Gene Clusters because changing the expression of a single gene is unlikely to significantly influence this balance. It is simply too little effort for too big a job. For example, can you imagine a goalkeeper in a soccer game being responsible both for scoring goals and defending the net, while playing against an entire team . . . by himself? No matter how great you make that goalkeeper, he or she cannot succeed.

IDENTIFY, TARGET, RESET

Now that we could **identify** these clusters of genes that were linked to aging—Youth Gene Clusters—the next and most important challenge for us was to **target** the exact genes that were "expressing themselves" with aging characteristics, so that we could influence them and **reset** them to express themselves as they used to do in a more youthful state.

Now let me remind you, when we talk about genes expressing themselves, or "genetic expression," we mean simply the way that genes communicate their instructions to the cell.

We consider youthful gene expression to be optimal gene expression, but to meet that goal requires a delicate balancing act. Gene expression is never on or off, and it also is not all up or all down. It is about balance, with the goal to achieve optimal levels as those seen in youth.

For example, some genes in your skin are responsible for producing collagen. During youth, these genes are up-regulated (or showing high expression), meaning they produce a lot of collagen. Conversely, collagenase is responsible for breaking down collagen so that it can be replaced with fresh new collagen. When we are young, this gene is down-regulated (or has low expression). Because the collagen gene is highly expressed and the collagenase is lowly expressed, the genes are perfectly balanced to give the collagen in your skin the highest quality, leaving you with fresh, young-looking skin.

As we age, this gene expression balance changes. Over time, the gene that produces collagenase increases its expression, and the gene that produces collagen lowers its expression, reversing the balance that gave the skin its fresh, youthful look. Instead, the increased collagenase breaks down collagen faster than it is replaced so that the skin structure begins to age.

The focus of ageLOC science was to understand how to reset those genes, or modulate their expression back to youthful expression, and regain the balance of youth. By understanding the gene expression of multiple genes, we can help restore the fine balance to maintain healthy, youthful tissue. This is a fundamental tenet of the ageLOC approach. (See heatmap on page 107.)

REMEMBER, IT IS WHAT YOU DO WITH YOUR GENES THAT COUNTS

We talked earlier about the fact that our genes are not our destiny. Our grandmothers were only partly right, aging is *in* the genes, but it's not *all* about our genes. It's about what we *do* with our genes, or gene expression, that has the greatest impact on how we age.

One of the best examples of this is a study done on identical twins. Identical twins have the *exact* same genes, but they often age in dramatically different ways as a result of differences in gene expression in response to lifestyle factors, including nutrition.

Essentially what we learned from these twins is that it is not the genes that you were born with, but what you do with them that counts. It is the choices you make in things like nutrition, exercise, antioxidant intake, smoking, stress levels, and supplementation that influence gene expression and therefore aging. As you can see in the picture from this study, these twins, while identical in genetic make-up, look remarkably different.

It is clearly evident that the gene expression is influenced by diet, environmental factors, and lifestyle choices because we know they have identical genes. It is also evident that gene expression profiles can be influenced by external factors. This led us to believe that if we could adequately influence the expression of the genes, we could impact the resulting aging process as well. In our proprietary process of discovering ingredients that can influence gene expression, we have the ability to produce effective ways to reset the gene expression profile and restore youthfulness.

ATTACKING AGING BOTH INSIDE AND OUT

Today, over 75 scientists and collaborators continue the vital work to identify specific functional Youth Gene Clusters that are responsible for youthful attributes not only in the skin, but in every part of our bodies, from the brain, to muscles, to the heart and other organs.

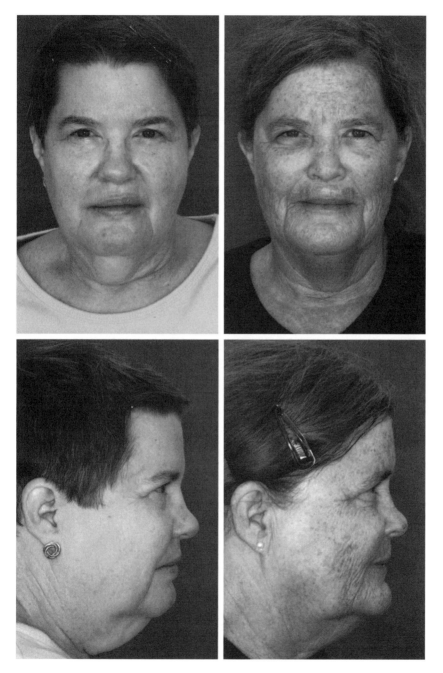

IDENTICAL TWINS AGE DIFFERENTLY.

Guyuren B et al. *Plast Reconstr Surg.* 2009 Apr; 123(4): 1321–31.

With our exclusive ability to "decode" the aging process using information based on our gene expression research, we believe we will be able to continually venture into new territory, making new, promising anti-aging discoveries.

We believe ageLOC is decades ahead of the pack in its ability to reset Youth Gene Clusters to behave more youthfully, helping to restore a more youthful balance in your body. This is extremely exciting. We are intent on using this science to help you look and feel better for the rest of your life—with good health and vigor. In all of my 30 years of research and development of innovative products, ageLOC technology is the most exciting to me in that it holds the greatest potential to help people of all ages live better lives, men and women alike.

DYING HEALTHY

As I stated in the last chapter, the goal is to "die young as late as possible." Our discoveries are referred to as anti-aging; actually, despite the use of this term, I am *not* against aging. What I *am* interested in is the science of maintaining health until you die.

Nobody minds getting older, but everyone minds looking older and less attractive and having their body feel old. We want to enjoy all the years of our lives, even as we age.

The paradox of age is that while we are young and able, we usually can't afford, and don't have the time to do what we would like to do. As we age, we become more financially capable and have more time to do what we want, but then we don't have the energy and vitality to do it.

I think George Bernard Shaw nailed it when he said, "Youth is wasted on the young!"

Well, the good news is, not anymore. With our discovery we understand how gene expression can help improve the way people age.

Our mission is to utilize our ageLOC understanding to help every single person on this planet live their life potential with maximum good looks, good health, and vitality. Over 750,000 independent distributors around the world are as passionate about this as I am because they have seen the results for themselves and desire to share it with others.

What does this look like? Whatever age you live to, be it 80, 90, or 100, you want to look and feel wonderful. You want to be able to walk, think, take care of yourself, and be independently vigorous all those years. I call this "youthspan."

YOUTHSPAN INDEX

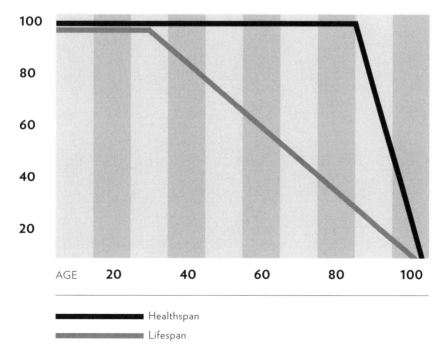

If you are living an unhealthy, unproductive life, what joy is there in that? Who would want to have their life extended under such circumstances? If your body is hard-wired to live only 80 years, your goal is undoubtedly to live it as well as possible.

That is my goal too, and with ageLOC you can.

"The great thing about getting older is that you don't lose all the other ages you've been."

MADELEINE L'ENGLE

I DEEPLY HOPE THAT BY NOW YOU ARE AS OPTIMISTIC AND energized as I am about looking and feeling younger for as long as you live. Consider these possibilities:

What if you won the "Back to the Future" award for looking the youngest at your high school reunion?

What if you could experience the fun of making people crazy wondering whether you had an extreme makeover?

What if you were faster than every bicyclist in the race, including those 10 years younger than you?

What if taking a nap in the middle of the day became a thing of the past?

What if you could live your life without the fear of being dependent on others?

What if you could help your ninth grader with his algebra without a cheat sheet?

What if you had more hits than you could handle on your eHarmony.com personal profile?

It should come as no surprise that I believe you can enjoy all these benefits with the science of ageLOC. It can be *the* solution in your struggle against the sources and signs of aging. We are going to help you look and feel better, outside and *in*!

THE AGING PROCESS

The film *City Slickers* takes a humorous look at the aging process. Three guys, friends in their late 30s, spend a couple of weeks each year going on "adventures," trying to convince themselves that they haven't lost their youth. They run with the bulls in Pamplona, go on sky diving vacations, etc. Finally, they go to a dude ranch in New Mexico to drive cattle.

In one of the first scenes of the film, Mitch Robbins, played by Billy Crystal, goes to speak to his 9-year-old son's class on career day. This also happens to be his 39th birthday and he's depressed.

He says something like the following:

When you're a teenager you think you can do anything—and you do.

20s are a blur.

30s? You raise your family.

40s? You grow a potbelly and music gets too loud.

50s? You have a minor surgery. You'll call it a procedure, but, it's a surgery.

60s? You'll have a major surgery. The music is still too loud but you can't hear it anyway.

70s? You retire, eat dinner at two, lunch around ten, and breakfast the night before.

80s? You'll have a major stroke and start babbling.....Any questions?

Okay. I'll admit it. I laughed. Yet, there is something so hauntingly possible about this scenario that it really isn't funny. Unless we impact the aging process, this breakdown could be *exactly* what happens to us.

BUT WHAT IF WE CAN CHANGE THE AGING PARADIGM?

My whole career, with all due respect to Billy Crystal, has been focused on answering this question—how can we ensure that the longer lives we now lead will be healthy and productive? What can I, as a scientist, do to make this happen?

As I've explained, in starting on this quest, my colleagues and I determined that the best way to demonstrate the power of ageLOC research was to focus first on the remarkable, beautiful organ, the skin. At the skin level, you can truly *see* the difference. This visual evidence makes it easy to understand that ageLOC science has translated into products that can elicit change with a meaningful benefit to the appearance of your skin.

So the next question to confront my team and me has been, "What about the *inside*?" Could the excellent results we've had in our research on Youth Gene Clusters relating to aging of the skin be replicated for other parts of the aging process affecting energy and good health? What if we could identify them and, as we've done with influencing the expression of the skin gene clusters, reset them as well?

The answer is yes. Once again, ageLOC has rounded the first turn before the competition has even left the starting gate.

GETTING UNDER YOUR SKIN

ageLOC science now extends far beyond the skin, providing a road map to lead us to healthier and more fulfilling lives. We are taking the next great leap in anti-aging, which is to take ageLOC inside. We are focusing on vitality and longevity because aging doesn't only happen to the skin; it happens inside us as well. Think about this. When was the last time you saw someone who was sick and, even though he didn't tell you, you could just see it? It may seem illogical that internal illness can affect your appearance, but your health on the inside is reflected on the outside. We are all a sum of our parts, visible or not, and ageLOC strives to help enhance the whole person so that you can feel as good as you look.

So, in addition to the ageLOC products we offer that reset Youth Gene Clusters and influence skin on the *outside* of your body, we have also discovered insights on how to influence Youth Gene Clusters that work on the *inside* as well. We have cracked open the gene "Instruction Manual" to the most vital functions of your body so you can take ageLOC inside.

THE INNER YOU

The two biggest complaints about getting older are **looking** older and **feeling** older. ageLOC has provided answers to questions on how science can influence the genetic expression profile required for skin to behave in a more youthful manner. I have seen ageLOC work. I know it works.

Now I'd like to talk about **feeling** younger and what it can mean for you.

We all know, of course, that time marches on, but that doesn't mean we want to feel time's effects; not at all! Part of feeling older is feeling that loss of vitality. I like the word "vitality" because it gives a good mental picture of the strength and energy needed to live a good, rewarding, happy, productive life. I think if we age prematurely, we lose vitality in multiple ways. Let's discuss three of them.

PHYSICALLY

Losing vitality in our physical bodies means we quickly lose endurance, stamina, and we easily fatigue. We notice that we are less able to respond to stress and we can't stay out all night and be fine the next day. This loss of vitality does not have to be inevitable as we age. We can influence our physical vitality so that we can continue to have the strength and endurance we had in our youth. There have been great examples of aging people throughout the years who have maintained their physical vitality. One of my personal favorites took place at the 64th Academy Awards in 1992, when Jack Palance, having just completed his 42nd year in films at age 73, got up on stage to accept the Oscar for Best Supporting Actor and easily did half-a-dozen one-handed pushups. Or, what about the great-grandmother who, according to the American Water Ski Association, was probably the oldest waterskier in the United States—at 87 years. Now this is the kind of physical vitality we can all enjoy.

MENTALLY

One of the greatest compliments given to an older person is, "She's still sharp as a tack!" I agree. Too often when people age mentally they lose sharpness, clarity, focus, memory, and alertness. This is the one that personally worries me the most.

I want to be like the great comedian Bob Hope who was still out there making jokes until he died at 100. Tragically, one of his best friends, Ronald Reagan, 40th President of the United States, died of Alzheimer's Disease. Universally considered to be one of the brightest political minds and great orators of our century, this brilliant man's intellect and intelligence died an untimely death 10 years before his body did at 93.

When you and I are 93, we should be able to read, imagine, invent, dream, and explain our ideas and philosophies to people eager to listen.

A colleague recently attended the funeral of her former piano teacher who died at 98. She was pleasantly shocked to discover that her dear mentor had taught piano into her 90s, racking up an impressive group of nearly 500 students. Imagine being able to live such an influential life for that many years. That's not all. The woman had suffered all her life from a severe form of polio. In spite of not being able to walk, she more than compensated with mental athleticism. Then there is Selma Plaut. She went back to school in her late 90s and received her bachelor's degree at 100 years young. It was reported that, upon her graduation, the local newspaper asked her what kind of degree she received. Her reply was, "History. I've lived most of it and I might as well get credit for it." Now this is the kind of mental vitality we can all enjoy.

SEXUALLY

Aging shouldn't mean that you don't live a full and complete life. It is common in today's scrambled and stressful world to have less time and less energy for sex. Both men and women want to feel that "get up and go" now and later in life.

For an extended length of time, usually up until age 40, women's bodies are incredibly powerful sexually in terms of the ability to create new life. But, eventually they go through a long and sometimes very exhausting period of menopause. Don't think you get to escape, men! Believe me, you go through "the change of life" to some degree. Some call it low testosterone. Others jokingly call it *man-o-pause*. For both sexes, there is inevitably some loss of sexual vitality as we age. I don't believe it has to happen. There is no reason for the light to dim in our love life.

MITOCHONDRIA: THE BODY'S POWER PLANTS

Given an optimal environment, our bodies are capable of creating all of the energy and vitality we need. It's our goal with ageLOC science to give the body all the help it needs. Let me explain to you where energy comes from.

The answer is food and oxygen.

Food affects us at the cellular level because our bodies have to convert the energy in the foods we eat into a form of energy that our cells can actually use. We convert that energy into adenosine triphosphate or ATP. This is analogous to the way we convert energy from coal into a form of energy we can use to power our homes, otherwise known as electricity. Just as we cannot plug our power cord into a block of coal, we cannot add food to our cells and expect them to run. Just as our cities have coal-fired power plants to generate electricity, our bodies too, have power plants called **mitochondria**. These tiny little power plants, located inside the cell, convert food into energy (ATP), which is in essence our cellular electricity—it fuels all our biological functions.

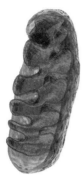

MITOCHONDRIA

YOUR MITOCHONDRIA DECREASE WITH AGE

Under normal conditions when we are young, our body functions receive plenty of energy. How often when we were in college or our early years working did we get up before dawn, gulp down a latte and a doughnut, spend the day in class or working, run five miles, party hearty or study into the wee hours of the morning, and then get up the next day to do it all again, without noticeably wearing down?

Then, sometime in our thirties or forties, usually depending on how hard we've pushed ourselves, our bodies begin to lose power. We feel a noticeable difference in energy and vitality because, over time, our mitochondrial efficiency begins to gradually decline and our bodies produce fewer and fewer mitochondria per cell. In essence, our body is supplying less energy, yet our bodies haven't slowed down! We still need just as much energy—if not more—especially for the brain, heart, and muscles.

It is not surprising that this happens. Think about it: our coal-fired power plants decline in efficiency as they age, too. It is the same concept. What do we do with our coal plants? We retrofit them with new technologies so that they work more efficiently, and we build new power plants so that each one does not have to work so hard. So how does this apply to our internal power plant, our mitochondria?

BOOSTING YOUR MITOCHONDRIA

There are certain things we can do, like aerobic exercise and consuming specific nutrients, that can stimulate our gene expression to produce building blocks for new mitochondria. Each stimulates the production of new mitochondria, as well as stimulating the repair of our existing mitochondria so that they operate more efficiently.

But more help is at hand.

DIAGRAM OF A CELL

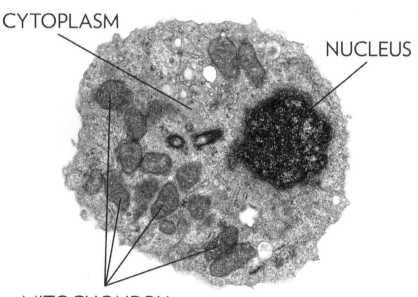

CYTOPLASM

NUCLEUS

MITOCHONDRIA

THE FLIP SIDE OF MITOCHONDRIA

The free radical theory of aging suggests that aging may result from, or at least be exacerbated by, the accumulation of molecular damage caused by free radicals. Free radicals have been associated with age-related diseases, including cancer, heart disease, diabetes, and Alzheimer's. Even in young, healthy people, substantial amounts of free radicals are generated inside a cell during mitochondrial-mediated cellular energy production. When the production of such free radicals exceeds the cells' radical quenching (antioxidant) capacity, excess free radicals cause damage to the cells, including the mitochondria. Such free radical damage to mitochondria accumulates over time and can impair metabolism and energy production, leading to cellular aging. The damage can also go beyond the mitochondria; free radicals in excess of the cells' antioxidant protection system can damage other cellular components, including DNA. In order to minimize free radical damage, antioxidants are an important part of an anti-aging regimen protecting against both mitochondrial and DNA damage.

Antioxidants, therefore, help protect cells in the body by neutralizing free radicals, and a powerful technology is available to measure antioxidants noninvasively in the body in order to help people monitor their antioxidant levels on a regular basis.

In 2009 our scientist team identified the first internal Youth Gene Cluster that comprises 52 genes tied to mitochondrial function. This is the Youth Gene Cluster related to mitochondria in the cells.

We started by focusing on three key tissues: the brain, heart, and muscles because they have the highest concentrations of mitochondria.

MITOCHONDRIAL YOUTH GENE CLUSTER & YOUTHFUL VITALITY

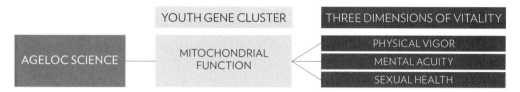

Our research team has now studied and tested the ingredients that specifically help the mitochondria Youth Gene Clusters and their production so that our cells have the energy to operate like they did when we were young.

To give you an idea of our research into these clusters, let me tell you about two mice. They have identical genetic coding. These two mice are living out their short lives (about 3 years which is actually about 96 years recalculated to human years). One mouse is fed a nutritionally complete mouse food. You wouldn't like it, but he does. The other mouse eats the same food except it includes an ingredient from our new ageLOC vitality formula that we hypothesized would reset the Youth Gene Clusters associated with the mitochondria in his cells.

At this writing, the mice are still alive. Sadly, the one who is only eating good food doesn't look very well at 96. He has nearly lost all of his strength and energy. He looks, frankly, old. The other, living on the same food fortified with the ageLOC ingredient, looks terrific.

The ageLOC mouse still has soft, silky fur, bright eyes, and plenty of energy to run around doing whatever laboratory mice do.

Such experiments are part of our ongoing work in identifying Youth Gene Clusters that are related to aging throughout our bodies. This research continues to reveal promising new areas for ageLOC, allowing us to pursue science that can help you age gracefully and with the strength and vitality of a younger you.

ALAS, EVEN AGELOC ISN'T ENOUGH

Obviously, I'm the first to discuss the amazing properties of ageLOC science. We are very proud of our work and hope to be able to help people all over the world look and feel younger.

But to maximize the power of our science, you need to do your part. There is a great quote by Mark Twain that says, "The only way to keep your health is to eat what you don't want, drink what you don't like, and do what you'd rather not." I love this quote because even though I don't agree with *exactly* what he says, I agree with the concept. To keep your health, *you* have to *do* something.

How well you age will be highly influenced by your lifestyle choices. There are a lot of factors that go into aging, many of which are related to *how* you live your life and *what* you do with your time. Let me give you a few examples:

— Just as the harmful effects of sleeplessness cannot be cured by the artificial buzz of caffeine overload, neither can any supplement replace vital REM sleep rejuvenation. Early to bed and early to rise is still good advice.

— You have to "mind" your brain to keep sharp-witted and clear thinking. Your brain needs stimulation and challenging thinking. Reading even just ten minutes a day, for example, can help to keep your brain active and sharp.

— Gorging on an excessive amount of calories, fat, and sugar adds weight and fat. Excess weight and excess fat can lead to health problems such as diabetes and heart disease that cannot be overcome by simply taking a supplement. Eating a healthy diet and getting daily exercise always has been and always will be a part of taking proper care of your body.

— You can't kid yourself into thinking a diet of energy bars and high sugar drinks is good nutrition and then expect a handful of even the best supplements to fill in the gap.

— You have to keep an eye on your vision by protecting your eyes from harmful sun rays and eating lots of dark-green, leafy vegetables.

I think you get the point. You need to decide, *are you worth the time to add quality time to your life?* Are you willing to make the effort to match the effort we have put into developing ageLOC products?

SAYING YES TO LIFE

Life is a gift we can't refuse.

Have you ever thought about that? Regardless of our birth experience or circumstances, we all made the miraculous journey. I truly believe that most people recognize their lives as extraordinary gifts and, like something rare and precious, they want to protect it.

More importantly, I think they are compelled to do it, which, I think is the main reason people are so fascinated by anti-aging. Beyond vanity, beyond narcissism, I believe we, as humans, are survivors.

GENES ARE SURVIVORS

Did you know that genes are survivors as well? In fact, they are eternal. I mean that in this sense: genes are inherently driven to duplicate themselves, reproduce, and pass their genetic information on. They came from our ancestors. They will survive into our progeny. Every single cell in our bodies is sustained by these amazing little survivors. And these little survivors, when given what they need (antioxidants, proper nutrition, sleep, supplementation, etc.), will do what they were meant to do.

SPIRIT OF SURVIVAL

World-renowned author Gail Sheehy, writer of *Passages, New Passages,* and *Understanding Men's Passages*—ground-breaking books on aging—wrote another remarkable book called *Spirit of Survival.* In 1981, while researching a news story on the Cambodian refugees, Sheehy interviewed an eleven-year-old girl whose family had been annihilated by the Pol Pot regime. From Mohn Phat's story, Sheehy extrapolates the characteristics of the incredible survival spirit she believes we all have, resilience, courage, fortitude, determination, ability to love, and many other qualities that help us endure just about any challenge.

The amazing story of another survivor, Aron Ralston, illustrates this. An experienced mountain climber, he was hiking alone in a remote desert in 2003 when a boulder dislodged and trapped him by the arm. For five days he survived with little water and no food, even drinking his own urine to survive. Finally, driven by an inner determination to survive, and summoning all of his courage, he leveraged his arm between two rocks, broke both the ulna and radius bones, and sawed through the soft flesh of his arm with a dull knife. Near death but even more determined to survive, he rappelled down a sheer 65-foot cliff and started walking out of the canyon in the hot, midday sun, eight miles to his vehicle. Luckily, he ran into a couple from the Netherlands who gave him water and two cookies, then notified authorities. He was rescued by helicopter and taken to safety. Today, he still climbs mountains, having invented a number of ingenious aids for one-armed climbers.

Now, I would personally never recommend climbing or any other outdoor adventure alone, so that you don't *have* to survive these kinds of situations, but the point is the same; we are a species built to survive!

LETTING AGELOC HELP YOU LIVE YOUR BEST LIFE

So what do these hallmarks of the victorious personality have to do with ageLOC? I think if we did enough research into our ancestors, who share our genetic code, we would discover that we have inherited a formidable spirit of survival through them.

People are born fighters. Babies endure hardship to be born and come out screaming to get on with life. They demand nurturing and proper sustenance without question.

While life's challenges beat some people into submission, I believe that for most of us this simple determination to live—and live well—endures even into adulthood.

In order to have great lives, **we have to demand for ourselves nurturing and proper sustenance without question.** We expect and work hard to have the best so that we can give our best. I unequivocally believe that in the skin and nutritional arena, ageLOC is simply the best science there is.

IF YOU COULD HAVE WHAT YOU WANT

If someone asked you what you think you would most want as you age into your 70s, 80s, and beyond, what would you say? As a person who has been involved in the health sciences nearly my entire life, I know what I would say. Good health. Without it, everything else loses its luster.

Let's say you amass a great fortune in your life. Well, that is wonderful, but if you aren't healthy enough to do anything, you will spend that fortune seeking for the one thing you lack—health. Or maybe you have a beautiful family with wonderful children and maybe even grandchildren. Can you really enjoy them if you don't have the health to participate in life with them? Wouldn't you want the vitality to enjoy them? Good health is simply critical to happiness, and because of that we need to fight hard, giving everything we have to get it.

In 1998, basketball legend Michael Jordan contracted the flu on the day of Game 6 of the National Basketball Association finals between his Chicago Bulls and the Utah Jazz. Jordan literally dragged himself out of bed to play. Game 6 was a tough battle for the two teams, and the Jazz had a lead late in the game. Down by three points, Jordan found some "superhuman" reserves to give the Bulls the final win. Jordan hit a driving layup to bring the Bulls within one, then stole the ball from Karl Malone and hit the game winning shot with 5.2 seconds remaining on the clock. The score was 87–86. He would be named the finals MVP for the sixth time in his career.

How did he do that? He recognized the critical importance of the situation so he was able to muster the strength, stamina, and fortitude to play even while sick.

That's part of what ageLOC is about! It is about helping us find the solutions to play well in our most important moments. ageLOC revitalizes the mitochondria, which return to us youthful vitality, helping us play the best "game" of life we possibly can. That's why I believe so strongly in ageLOC.

AGELOC'S GIFT

ageLOC is all about giving you a fighting chance at having more youthful, vigorous bodies to enjoy better days, weeks, months, and years. The kind of existence you create with that gift is what you are all about.

Death Becomes Her is an excellent allegorical film about aging. Two gorgeous women, played by Goldie Hawn and Meryl Streep, are rivals for one man's affections. The hapless dupe, played by Bruce Willis, also just happens to be a famous plastic surgeon. Could it be that he is just a pawn in their never-ending quest to get ahead of the relentless ravages of time? These women live their lives for pure vanity, but, realizing that even he can't sculpt them in a never-ending makeover, the women make a desperate pact with the devil (in this case, a beautiful goddess). They want eternal life. They get it. Sort of. They should have read their Greek mythology. This is something like the case of Eos and Tithonus but with an even more cruel twist. They are not really given eternal life. They are just "undead."

It's a terrifying black comedy. I say that because even when I laugh at some of the most creative sight gags ever produced in a film (Picture Meryl Streep mincing along in evening gown and spike heels, looking gorgeous, except for one tiny flaw: her head is screwed on backward!), I wonder if some people still get this all wrong, like the two vain women. Anti-aging is not about vanity. Now you may look better and you can certainly feel better, and while you can bask in both of those, your greatest pleasures will come in life itself and the new opportunities and longevity that can open up to you.

WHAT'S ON YOUR BUCKET LIST?

My work in anti-aging provides human beings unprecedented opportunity for good health and well-being until the day they die. Do you look forward to love, service, family, learning, security, and the time to do what you have always wanted to do? These are all good things, wonderful things, but without good health inside and out, try enjoying any of them.

Do you have a "bucket list"? A list of things you have always wanted to do? Intend to do? Even some things that you only dream might be possible? There is probably not one thing on your list that poor health or looking decrepit wouldn't put a huge damper on.

JOE'S BUCKET LIST

Let me tell you that way up near the top of my bucket list is exactly what I am doing right now. With ageLOC, I am fulfilling one of my professional and personal goals to develop the science that can help every person on earth live a healthier life. Not just that. I want people to die healthy. I want them to live their lives to their maximum potential.

This is not entirely selfless. I have a big bucket, and I want to get to the bottom of it before I die. Of course I want to see both of my sons, Colin and Christopher, fulfill their careers and dreams. I want to live a very long life with my wife, Ping. When we are both 80, I'd like to hold her hand and skydive out of an airplane!

Okay, even ageLOC can't guarantee that all of our dreams will come true!

No matter. Having great, healthy skin and a strong, healthy body with organs running at top efficiency makes the prospect of a long life a whole lot more appealing. I live my life today so that my tomorrows—and yours—are ones that can be lived at their best. Like Oprah Winfrey's famous mantra, I would like us all to be able to "live our best life."

"The great enemy of the truth is very often not the lie, deliberate, contrived, and dishonest, but the myth, persistent, persuasive, and unrealistic."

JOHN F. KENNEDY

THERE ARE MANY OPTIONS AVAILABLE TO COMBAT THE signs and symptoms of aging both outside and inside the body, but not all are created equal. In this chapter we will discuss some of the trends that I see in the anti-aging industry.

TODAY'S ANTI-AGING CLAIMS

For every scientific discovery or discussion out there on aging, there are as many debates about how to approach the aging issue. In fact, there are a lot of outrageous anti-aging "solutions" being hocked out there in the private sector. My growing frustration is that many people see the benefits but don't always adequately weigh the risks. One of my motivations in writing this book is to counter some of these misleading claims and misinformation. You will be able to use this knowledge to improve your own health and well-being and share your knowledge with others also interested in aging well. As the famous Roman writer and thinker Cicero said about acquiring knowledge, if it is to be useful "it must have the fullest possible supply of facts."

NOT ALL PRODUCTS ARE EQUAL

There are many stakeholders in the anti-aging market: those who invent the products, those who market the products, and the consumers who purchase them. The list is long, including drug and supplement companies, cosmetic companies, pharmaceutical and healthcare companies, biotech companies, and nutrition companies. All of them are involved in the various aspects of this huge business, from manufacturers, retailers and super retailers, technology providers, research and development (R&D) companies, to universities.

This is an awesome array of people spending billions of dollars in pursuit of youth and beauty. Admittedly, I am one of those stakeholders, but I assure you that my days in Pharmanex taught me not all products are equal. Actually, few so-called anti-aging experts have the insight into the real remedies of aging because they simply do not have the latest science, the knowledge, or the commitment to make a high-quality product. Just because a marketing department hangs a shingle on a company saying "Anti-Aging Experts" does not make it so. It's about as logical as saying that being able to boil an egg makes me an expert chef.

MEGATRENDS FOR YOUTH SEEKERS

Due to the pressures people feel to look younger, far too many are being persuaded that their only real anti-aging defense is to resort to any number of invasive procedures or risky surgeries.

Unfortunately, the decision to jump into using such methods is often an unnecessary overreaction to the pervasive feeling of helplessness people have when they are confronted with the signs of aging.

As a scientist, it greatly disturbs me how cavalier some people are about putting their own bodies at risk. Look at this "Coupon of the Week" ad that came across my computer screen:

A little bird told us that when you get older, unexpected lines and wrinkles appear on your face. Say goodbye to crow's feet and other pesky lines with today's deal: Get 20 units of Botox for anywhere on your face at (company name withheld) for $149 (regularly $300). Botox, a protein injected into your problem areas with a tiny needle, can scare away those crow's feet as well as the lines between your brows and across your forehead—something to smile about with the threat of aging flying over you. While the intrusion to your face is as light as a feather, the results are dramatic and lasting. Don't wait for others to egg you on; swoop into the clinic today and really give them something to crow about.

I actually wanted to laugh. However, if I had the procedure done, I wouldn't be able to laugh. Botulinum toxin works by blocking the chemical signal from the nerve that causes the muscle to contract. The result is minimized movement of specific muscles in the face and neck—a blank expression with very little to smile about.

COSMETIC SURGICAL PROCEDURES	% CHANGE
BREAST AUGMENTATION	+48%
TUMMY TUCK	+89%

COSMETIC MINIMALLY INVASIVE PROCEDURES	% CHANGE
BOTOX	+1266%
SOFT TISSUE FILLERS	+469%

American Society of Plastic Surgeons 2010 Report

BE WARY OF INVASIVE COSMETIC SOLUTIONS

What about collagen injections? Facial surgery? These procedures utilize needles, knives, and staples, stretching of the face, trimming off excess flesh, stitching, scarring, bruising—this is the frightening reality of facelift surgery.

Regardless of what the slick advertising and glossy brochures may say about these procedures being wonderful for anti-aging, they are temporary, expensive, and invasive options that do not bring lasting results.

I'm not here to criticize surgeons. I've worked in the medical field all my life and know that most of the surgeons who perform facial surgery are highly trained, highly principled, and very good at what they do. When horrific accidents or unfortunate birth defects occur, their skilled work saves lives. Facial reconstruction and plastic surgery have created miracles for millions of deformed individuals. Witness the Operation Smile doctors and nurses who, donating their time and talents, repair cleft lips and palates that normally ruin children's lives all over the world. Burn patients *require* these types of procedures not only for their cosmetic benefit, but for survival.

But many facial surgeries are performed as cosmetic solutions to counteract the appearance of aging. According to the American Academy of Plastic Surgery, the top three surgical invasive procedures are breast implants, liposuction, and facelifts. Facelifts can cost $10,000 to $20,000, depending on the amount of surgery performed and the reputation of the plastic surgeon.

Common sense would have to tell you that invasive procedures inevitably carry some risk. The high cost, pain, and extended recovery time can turn out to be more than you bargained for. The decision to undergo surgery should not be taken lightly.

A BETTER WAY

If we give them a chance, our bodies are remarkably intuitive, capable at a cellular level of repairing themselves.

I can say this with full confidence based on my work with ageLOC, which has gone beyond other companies in understanding aging at

RISKS OF PLASTIC SURGERY

Any surgery, including cosmetic procedures like plastic surgery, has inherent risks—whether expected scars or an unexpected fatality. Anyone considering elective plastic surgery should be aware of the potential dangers.

One of the most common complications from plastic surgery is scarring. While most surgeons will try to hide the incision, patients will still end up with permanent scarring. Unsightly scarring can result in the need for additional surgeries.

Infection at the point of incision is another common risk. Infection can worsen scarring and prolong recovery.

One of the more serious risks is numbness, tingling, or muscle function that can occur from nerve damage and may be permanent.

While everyone has some inherent risks, people with a history of cardiovascular disease, diabetes, or obesity have much higher risk of complications.

American Society of Plastic Surgeons

the cellular and genetic level. Our science is based on the discovery of internal sources of aging that contribute to how we look and feel as we age. Most aging signs are the result of slowed normal skin cell function, sometimes as a result of environmental damage, sometimes in the way genes are expressed. The information in this book can help you choose a better way to look younger.

LOOKING GOOD IS ONLY HALF OF THE EQUATION

As much as people want to look younger than their years, they also want to return to the youthful energy and vitality of their younger years. In a consumer survey conducted in 20 countries, 63% of respondents stated that they "are highly attentive toward their health." This is indicative of consumers globally taking more responsibility for their health.

Here, too, though, quick fixes seem very appealing but are far from the healthiest way to maintaining vigor.

CONSIDER THIS

The global health and wellness market brought in $569 billion in 2008. That's a lot of people wanting to know how they can make their lives more healthy and look and feel great while doing it.

Global OTC Healthcare, July 2009.

YOU CAN'T DRINK YOUR WAY TO HIGH ENERGY

While some people embrace invasive surgical procedures to improve their outside appearance, others chug down energy drinks to feel better on the inside. Seeking to regain lost vitality, millions turn to energy "boost" drinks and energy bars that are so filled with sugar, fats, carbohydrates, and stimulants that it's a wonder these products don't literally fly off the shelves by themselves.

What users don't often understand is that the boost of energy obtained from these drinks is the result of a stimulant effect, not real energy. The effects are only temporary and often result in an energy "crash" that can last a lot longer than the high.

Most of these products are loaded with empty calories (sugar), salt, caffeine (one very high-potency energy drink has 505 mg of caffeine, compared to a standard 12-ounce can of cola which has 35 mg of caffeine), or guarana, an herb that is full of caffeine and allows consumers to think they are getting their caffeine boost "naturally." Caffeine is a stimulant that works through the central nervous system. Too much caffeine can lead to nervousness, anxiety, and irritability. Since it is a stimulant, the perceived energy derived from caffeine is temporary, usually leading to a crash after a few hours, requiring more intake of caffeine. Too late in the day, this cycle of caffeine intake to combat fatigue can lead to sleep disruption. A poor night's sleep means more caffeine the following day, and the vicious cycle is perpetuated. Some of the same issues occur with sugar intake. A big, sweet soda fulfills the need for short-term energy, followed by a big crash, not to mention the calorie overload that comes with sugary drinks and snacks.

Too many young people are drinking energy drinks *like they should be drinking water* because neither they nor their parents understand the risks involved. Athletes as well are drinking energy drinks thinking they enhance performance. Many well-known, high-potency energy drinks have already been banned in Europe due to the fact that, after consuming them, several athletes have died from severe dehydration during exercise or training.

Why am I so concerned about these drinks? Because for the most part, they are useless in terms of creating authentic energy and, when abused, can be risky.

RISKS OF ENERGY DRINKS

Energy drinks only produce a temporary stimulant "high," which often results in a dramatic "low."

When consumed by those with diabetes, hypoglycemia, and heart conditions, energy drinks may exacerbate the condition.

Younger people under the age of 18 should not use energy drinks at all. In this age group the effects of caffeine are dramatically increased, causing kids to "bounce off the walls."

An increased level of caffeine in the body can lead to stomach problems, panic attacks, anxiety, and cardiac arrhythmias. Caffeine is also known to mask the symptoms of fatigue. When symptoms of fatigue are not apparent, the body is already overworked while the person is continuing activity, which puts further strain on the heart.

Stimulants in energy drinks (for example guarana, yohimbine HCL, evodiamine, yerba-mate, N-Acetyl-L-Tyrosine, and others) have similar effects on the brain's neurotransmitters—dopamine, serotonin, and epinephrine—as drugs of abuse. Adolescents and young adults are more vulnerable to addictions because their memory and reward centers in their brains are underdeveloped.

Energy drinks contain dehydrating agents which can severely lower fluid levels in the body.

Using energy drinks with alcohol is a double whammy. When you mix the two, you are mixing caffeine, which is a stimulant and speeds up the central nervous system, and alcohol, a depressant which does the complete opposite. Basically, mixing these two drinks is like getting into your car and having one foot on the brake and one on the gas at the same time. Some energy drinks contain alcohol. Alcoholic energy drinks are often sold in cans that are poorly labeled, resembling nonalcoholic beverages.

See References in Appendix

YOU HAVE MUCH BETTER CHOICES

In the fight to retain your youthfulness, resorting to invasive practices, temporary fixes, and stimulant use should be your last ditch effort—not your first solution.

With ageLOC, we know that vitality is found at the cellular level and can be accessed in several ways. A large part of my mission with ageLOC is to provide the kind of supplementation that belies any need or desire for such artificial stimulants.

THE MYTH BUSTER

As I stated at the beginning of this chapter, for every discovery or *great* thing in the anti-aging arena, a "not-so-great" item emerges. These "myths," as I like to call them, need to be debunked.

Let me bust a few myths for you right now, the first one being that we claim that ageLOC science is an alternative to medical practices.

ageLOC is something entirely different in that we focus on genes, and natural supplemental support for influencing gene expression. We believe in prevention. We believe in supporting the body's natural youthful mechanisms.

Myth: You have to accept what you inherit from your parents, like wrinkles or crow's-feet.

Fact: Debunking this falsehood is perhaps our most important breakthrough. While you do have to accept your parents' genetic coding, you are not stuck with your parents' **gene expression. That you can influence.**

ZOE DRAELOS, MD., Dermatologist and Editor-in-Chief, *Journal of Cosmetic Dermatology*

Myth: *Aging spots are inherited.*

Fact: Although your unique genetic composition determines how dark or light your skin can be, the development of age spots is caused by increased numbers of melanocytes in your skin. These melanocytes are cells that produce high levels of melanin, which results in a specific area of hyperpigmentation on the skin's surface. Although lentigenes, or brown-pigmented spots, may develop slowly over time or appear suddenly on the skin, they are most likely the result of long-term exposure to sunlight over many years. Protection from UV light is the best way to prevent these skin pigmentation cells from adopting a gene expression that would cause them to produce more pigment in localized areas, forming brown spots.

BRYAN FULLER, PH.D., Adjunct Professor Department of Dermatology, University of Oklahoma Health Sciences Center

Myth: *Sensitive skin is caused by bad genes.*

Fact: While your genetic makeup defines individual uniqueness, the expression of your genes is what is most important. While it is true that certain individuals have skin that is more sensitive to a variety of substances—chemicals, allergens, etc.—the skin's sensitivity response can be managed through a modified response to a skin "sensitizer." By reducing the level of an inflammatory response to a potential "sensitizer"—like an allergen or chemical irritant—the level of skin sensitivity can be significantly reduced.

HELEN KNAGGS, PH.D., Vice President, Global R&D, Nu Skin

Myth: Adjusting my "genes" to a youthful expression is extremely costly and requires specialized physicians and multiple doctor visits.

Fact: If your understanding is that the DNA code is fixed for life, you'd be quite right. Even though there is a constant cycle of damage and repair to the DNA over the course of our lives, our DNA basically does not change. That's why I'm not surprised that there's a common misunderstanding (probably reinforced by our exposure to Marvel Comics' superhero characters) that any changes to our physical characteristics that are in any way attributable to our genes must necessarily involve some sort of genetic engineering, or changes to the actual structure of our genes.

Sure, to adjust our genes by using a genetic engineering or gene-splicing approach would be highly invasive, experimental, and expensive. But that's an approach reserved for the future and for diseased states.

In contrast, we now understand that the expression of our DNA—the translation of our DNA to a message that affects the biochemistry and behavior of the cell and ultimately the body—does change as we age. And that expression is also susceptible to being influenced by lifestyle and nutritional factors. This is a natural and helpful way to take the new view that we do have control over the direction and destiny of our wellness. I believe that one of the biggest genetic breakthroughs of our generation is the ability to measure the work output of our genes, and therefore to measure the effects of various natural ingredients to determine which are most helpful in obtaining that youthful expression pattern.

MARK BARTLETT, PH.D., Vice President, Global R&D, Pharmanex

Myth: I don't want to live past 65 because my parents did and seemed to get frail and inactive, and so it seems inevitable that I will become frail and inactive.

Fact: The chorus of a favorite rock song of mine goes as follows: "Now he's too old to rock 'n' roll, but he's too young to die" (from "Too Old To Rock 'n' Roll: Too Young To Die," Jethro Tull).

As children and as youth, most of us thought we'd live forever. We were also probably reminded from an early age how we had our father's nose and our mother's temperament. It's not surprising then, as we witnessed our parents and grandparents beginning to age, that we revisited our goals for immortality. Certainly none of us wants to find ourselves in that space between too old to enjoy life and too young to die, but it's a very limiting view to pin our destiny entirely on our genetic makeup passed down from mom and dad.

Again, though our genetic code is fixed for life, the code is only part of the story of who we are and where we're headed. Since the year 2002, the entire human genome has been sequenced, and science is now uncovering the secrets of how our genetic code expresses itself as a function of our diet and lifestyle. We are now standing on the precipice of a new paradigm, one that allows us to see more clearly that our genes are not our only destiny. We just need to learn the secrets of how to nudge our genes into expressing themselves in a healthy longevity pattern. But we need to start now. If we wait until we're 65 years old before we take control, then this myth may be self-fulfilling.

MARK BARTLETT, PH.D., Vice President, Global R&D, Pharmanex

Myth: The rate at which you get wrinkles is completely dependent on your genetics.

Fact: It's what we do with what we have (genes) that gives us wrinkles. Sun exposure, oxidative stress, repeated facial motions all contribute to the formation of wrinkles. How many people have wrinkles on their buttocks? None. So, it's not the genes; it's what we do with the genes that we have. The way we direct the expression of our genes by our behavior is how we get or avoid developing wrinkles.

DALE KERN, Senior Scientist, Nu Skin

Myth: There is a single youth gene related to all aspects of aging.

Fact: Aging is a complex process that is likely to be impacted by multiple genetic and biochemical pathways. This complexity is underscored by the fact that hundreds of genes are involved in critical processes associated with aging, such as DNA repair, protein repair and turnover, and mitochondrial or energy metabolism. Gene expression profiling studies have shown that thousands of genes are likely to be involved in aging.

TOM PROLLA, PH.D., Co-Founder, LifeGen Technologies

Myth: It's impossible to identify the sources of aging.

Fact: Genetic studies in simple organisms, as well as similar studies in mammals, have begun to identify the key pathways that control aging. By understanding the biochemical functions associated with such pathways we can identify the sources of aging. Our growing understanding of the sources of aging is unprecedented and is leading to a revolution in how we intervene in the aging process.

TOM PROLLA, PH.D., Co-Founder, LifeGen Technologies

Myth: *It's impossible to measure aging at the genetic level.*

Fact: We have developed and patented technology that allows measurement of the aging process at the genetic (gene expression) level in individual organs, such as the brain, heart, skin, and muscle. This technology makes use of gene chips, a revolutionary technology that allows for the simultaneous analysis of gene activity of thousands of genes. Such technology allows us to identify compounds that impact aging by retarding its progression or even reversing it in some cases.

TOM PROLLA, PH.D. AND RICHARD WEINDRUCH, PH.D.,
Co-Founders, LifeGen Technologies

Myth: *Nutrients can't affect the way genes are expressed.*

Fact: The classical experiment in aging research, made more than 75 years ago in 1935 by Clyde McKay, reported a remarkable lifespan extension in rodents fed a calorie restricted diet. Since 1935, extending lifespan by calorie restriction has been observed in yeast, worms, flies, mice, dogs, nonhuman primates, and other species. It is generally believed in the scientific community that this will eventually also be proven in humans. All these studies convincingly show that nutrients affect the way genes are expressed.

Furthermore, nutrients in the diet, supplemented or provided topically, also affect how genes are expressed. Gene expression is controlled by enzymes that add or remove methyl groups to DNA or acetyl groups to proteins known as histones, that are wrapped around DNA, thereby activating or deactivating gene activity. Choline and folic acid are dietary sources of methyl groups; fat in the diet is a source of acetyl groups. If the diet is deficient in these nutrients, abnormal development may occur. What is very important is that such changes in gene activity can be retained throughout life and often for several generations affecting our offspring. This fast-growing research area is known as epigenetics.

LESTER PACKER, PH.D., Adjunct Professor, Department of Pharmacology and Pharmaceutical Sciences, University of Southern California

Myth: Once you reset your youthful gene expression you don't have to keep maintaining that expression.

Fact: Altering gene expression patterns with nutritional formulations is a reversible process since it does not lead to any direct change in our genome. In other words, it is the activity of the genes that is changed as opposed to any permanent change in gene (DNA) structure. Although this underlies the safety of such interventions, it also implies that changes are reversible and that continued supplementation is needed to maintain youthful gene expression patterns. Some changes in gene expression may revert back to a "normal" aged pattern in a few days after stopping supplementation, while others may take weeks or months to revert to their aged pattern. But eventually, all changes will revert back to the aged pattern if supplementation ceases. Importantly, retardation of aging will also stop once the formulations are no longer consumed, and this will compromise the long-term effectiveness of such supplementation strategies. For effective anti-aging intervention, supplementation should be started as early in adult life as possible and should be continued with minimal interruption. As the technology evolves, novel and even more powerful formulations will be developed, with increasing effectiveness, so users of this technology can "upgrade" their supplementation programs.

TOM PROLLA, PH.D., Co-Founder, LifeGen Technologies

Myth: Aging is dependent solely on environmental factors.

Fact: Aging is associated with a general decline in health; environmental factors, such as pollution, exposure to chemicals, alcohol, and smoking, can lead to age-related diseases. The major sources of aging are the result of endogenous factors. As a result of our daily activities, we consume oxygen and metabolize food. Over time, our energy factories (mitochondria) become less functional. Other parts of the cell that engage in high levels of activity, such as the nucleus, also suffer damage, and functional alterations in gene expression ensue. These multiple endogenous sources of aging are likely to operate in multiple tissues, but the contribution to each tissue is different. One of the long-term effects of endogenous sources of aging is alterations in gene expression patterns and resulting cellular dysfunction.

TOM PROLLA, PH.D., Co-Founder, LifeGen Technologies

JUST THE FACTS

So let's get out of the myths and the discussions and just state some facts for a moment.

Fact: My associates and I, in partnership with some of the most brilliant research teams in the world, are combining resources to understand the ultimate sources of aging.

Fact: We have found key sources of aging.

Fact: *You* can do something about all of these aging challenges because *we* have done something.

5

"It is health that is real wealth and not pieces of gold and silver."

MAHATMA GANDHI

I HAVE DISCUSSED THAT WE ARE INDEED AGING AND THAT we will continue to age. We know that there are many solutions out there to combat the signs of aging, some good—some not. We also know that we will probably live longer than our parents. Our children will probably live longer than we will. **So, naturally, we all have an enormous interest in reversing the appearance of aging and even slowing the negative aspects of the aging process inside our bodies!** Given that we are going to live longer, we want to look and feel better, longer. We demand it.

But why? Why do we care so much? Why *should* we care? Are we just a vain and selfish society? I don't think so. The aging process is very real and so is its impact on our lives. To give you just one example, in the 1920s the average life expectancy for an American male was

62 years old. The federal government set the retirement age at 65 years old, so, in other words, most people were working until they died! This is not the case anymore. When we retire now, we still have another life ahead of us. As a matter of fact, some people will even live long enough that their working years are actually shorter than their retirement years. I think there are a number of areas in our lives where looking and feeling younger are not just something we would like, but in this world . . . an absolute must.

WE NEED TO LOOK VITAL

With increased lifespan and decreased economic stability, many of us need to work well into our later years. If life asks us to keep working into our 70s and 80s, we want to have the ambition and genius to succeed and we want people to be confident we have them!

Take Craig, for instance, an intelligent, educated man in his late 50s who suddenly found himself, along with hundreds of thousands of others, out of a job in the economic downturn of 2008–2010. With an impressive resume yards long and experience that no college degree could possibly grant, he still found it difficult to find another job.

Why? Because in spite of the fact that people are now productive long beyond their 50s, society is **image-prejudiced**. This isn't just about looking older, it is about how you "present" yourself, both with your looks and your vitality. I sympathize with the many thousands facing this kind of prejudice. However, we live in the real world, and here are some real world truths: "older" skin looks less healthy, less vital, and less happy. Older skin creates the image of being tired and used up. It's thinner, less vibrant, and less radiant. Sagging muscles make a face look tired and ragged.

That's not all. Sagging muscles in our bodies and "tired" organs show up in our posture, bearing, and self-confidence. If we "feel" tired, we "look" tired. People don't want tired and run-down individuals working for their companies, they want energetic, youthful types who can put in the hours necessary and look like they have the stamina to fight the challenges that come in a positive and engaging way.

Like it or not, the perception that drives business is that youth is power. Youth is intelligence. Youth is vitality. That's why a 55-year-old who wants to be hired needs to look 40.

WE WANT TO BE PRODUCTIVE

Some of us have the financial means to retire but don't want to because we enjoy the challenge and we thrive on being productive. Robert is an acquaintance of mine who turned 65 ten years ago and has retired twice but keeps going right back to work! For him, retirement now means not *needing* to work, but he has found that he loves it! He finds retirement boring because he would rather be building something new than remembering something he built previously.

Other people don't even know the meaning of "retire." At age 65, "Colonel" Harland Sanders lost his family restaurant, took his first Social Security check of $105, and started peddling his Kentucky Fried Chicken recipe to potential franchisees. When Sanders finally died at 90, KFC® was a worldwide fast food phenomenon.

Margaret Mead, the famous cultural anthropologist, worked into her 70s, and Anna Mary Robertson Moses, better known as "Grandma Moses," started painting in her 70s and created over 3600 canvases in three decades. She died at 101.

Like these great individuals, many of us *want* to continue to be productive. We want the vitality and stamina to take advantage of our wisdom that comes through the years. We enjoy challenges, and we like the rigor and rhythm we have established by working hard for something greater in our lives.

TOP ACTIVITIES FOR THE AGING DEMOGRAPHIC

A recent survey conducted by the ProMatura Group, Pulte Homes, Inc., and Del Webb Communities shows that active recreation, especially adventurous pursuits, joins mainstays such as golf and tennis as top interests for older Americans. The list includes things like rollerblading, skiing, hiking, river rafting, kayaking, and hang gliding, as well as team sports like softball.

TOP SPORTS, ATHLETIC, AND OUTDOOR ADVENTURE PURSUITS

Activity	Percent ranked "extremely important"
SWIMMING	55.2%
GOLF	49.2%
BOWLING	34.4%
FISHING	30.1%
CANOEING/KAYAKING	26.2%

INCREASING IN POPULARITY

HIKING/CLIMBING/RAPPELLING	18.0%
RIVER RAFTING	17.8%
DOWNHILL SKIING	9.1%
ROLLERBLADING	7.3%
COMPETITIVE RUNNING	6.1%
HANG GLIDING/PARASAILING/PARACHUTING	6.0%

The aging demographic also wants to stay in shape. Working out remains a top priority, including walking and cardiovascular equipment workouts (treadmills, etc.) and training programs such as Pilates, tai chi, and yoga.

TOP HEALTH AND FITNESS PURSUITS

Activity	Percent ranked "extremely important"
WALKING	82.0%
CARDIOVASCULAR EQUIPMENT WORKOUTS	78.8%
STRENGTH/WEIGHT TRAINING EQUIPMENT WORKOUTS	67.4%
WATER AEROBICS EXERCISE CLASSES/WATER-BASED FITNESS	63.0%
SWIMMING	62.5%

INCREASING IN POPULARITY

BIKING	56.7%
BALANCE TRAINING PROGRAMS (YOGA, TAI CHI, PILATES)	51.3%
PERSONAL TRAINING	41.8%
SPINNING	18.1%

Although the trend is toward more active recreational opportunities, passive, brainy, creative, and technology options also show up as extremely important.

TOP CRAFTS AND CULTURAL ART PURSUITS

Activity	Percent ranked "extremely important"
CERAMICS/POTTERY/CLAY WORKS	28.4%
PAINTING AND DRAWING	27.2%
WOODCRAFTING	27.1%
STAINED-GLASS MAKING	26.9%
KNITTING	22.8%

TOP MEDIA AND TECHNOLOGY PURSUITS

Activity	Percent ranked "extremely important"
COMPUTER TECHNOLOGY—GENERAL	44.4%
PHOTOGRAPHY	33.5%
COMPUTER GRAPHICS	33.2%
DESKTOP PUBLISHING	27.6%
TELEVISON/CABLE TV PROGRAMMING	25.7%

http://www.seniorjournal.com

If your desire is to work, to be productive, to build something more for yourself and your loved ones, then we want that to be a reality for you for as long as possible.

WE WANT TO PLAY

Perhaps we are comfortable retiring and leaving work behind, but if we have more time in our later years for sports or recreation, we want to have the strength and stamina to do it and enjoy it.

The world was amazed when swimmer Dara Torres won her twelfth medal in the 2008 Olympics at the age of 41. This American mother from Florida had set dozens of world swimming records, even after having had reconstruction surgery on her knee. She is the first, and oldest, American swimmer to compete in five Olympic Games and, as of this writing, is preparing for a sixth. When asked about her age she said, "The water doesn't know what age you are."

Whether we are competing in a sport or simply participating for sheer enjoyment, we want the ability to play to our top capacity.

WE WANT MEMORIES

Longer lives for us and longer lives for our children mean we are probably going to live long enough to know our grandchildren and even our great-grandchildren. If life affords us this opportunity, then we want to have the brain capacity to remember them. We want the memories of a great and long life to remain with us and be vivid in our minds. We want the capacity to truly recall great moments so that we can relive them through the years.

We also want our posterity to know us as viable, intelligent, significant people who made a definite, positive contribution to their lives. We want them to be able to come to us for advice, call us with great news, and even just talk with us when they need a listening ear. We want to be a positive memory to them. But perhaps most of all, we don't want to end up as burdens to them. We do not want them forced to care for us because we didn't take good enough care of ourselves.

A VESTED INTEREST

We all have a vested interest in anti-aging. We all know stories of marvelous people who live as youthfully as the spirits inside of them. We all want this "old man strength" and vitality. Perhaps we don't want to work until we're 88, but if we're honest, we want to live as long as we're meant to live to the fullest of our capacity. It's interesting that outrageous amounts of money, time, and medical resources are expended on our bodies *after* they have been hit by age. What about throwing the same kind of resources at really effective measures for prevention? This isn't about vanity and selfishness. This is about looking and feeling great so that we can truly live our lives to the fullest.

Stephen R. Covey, author of *The Seven Habits of Highly Effective People*, proposes that we want to "live, love, learn and leave a legacy." We can't do this if we are just struggling to survive. If we don't have the physical, mental, and emotional capacity to thrive in life.

Incidentally, Covey himself is in his late seventies and is still a powerhouse writer and lecturer. I believe his credo is true of most people. It certainly is true of me. That's why I do the work that I do.

"And in the end it's not the years in your life that count. It's the life in your years."

ABRAHAM LINCOLN

EACH YEAR I TRAVEL OVER 200,000 MILES SPEAKING TO tens of thousands of people in presentations and seminars around the world. Inevitably, I am asked a lot of questions in these meetings about our science and our discoveries, and how they can benefit them personally. Since many of these questions seem to be frequent and universal, I thought I would take a moment to share my thoughts on these questions.

QUESTION:

While visiting in Singapore recently, an elderly, elegant woman asked me why she had "crow's-feet."

I said, "What do you mean, why?"

She explained that generations of women in her family have always taken pride in the fact that their faces never show any obvious signs of aging until well into their late 70s, yet here she was in her early 60s with crow's feet and she wanted to know why. Why can't I age like my mother?

ANSWER:

The answer to her question also addresses a lot of other questions about common concerns of aging such as wrinkles, age spots, sagging skin, and the like. Whether you *want* to age like your ancestors, or you *do not* want to age like your ancestors, the answer lies in the same understanding.

We start by learning a little more about her, and her environment. While most of her family lived out in the country, she lived in the city and had a very stressful job. She had a lot of sun damage when she was a child. Her diet had changed and she smokes. It was becoming clear that somehow her genes were influenced in a negative way by her environment and lifestyle.

But then I gave her the good news that she could do something to reduce the signs of aging. Her aging is in her own hands. She can begin by improving the factors around her by being more careful when in the sun, controlling stress, and improving her diet and exercise. I also informed her that her mother had good genes, and so does she. She can also improve her aging by resetting her aging sources. Remember, in ageLOC science parlance, we call these sources Youth Gene Clusters, and how these are expressed makes all the difference in the world in terms of how you age.

QUESTION:

Of course, that led to another question I get asked a lot: What does *"resetting"* Youth Gene Clusters mean?

ANSWER:

When we say we're going to *reset* Youth Gene Clusters, we're talking about restoring the fine balance that exists among aging-related genes in terms of their gene expression. In other words, each gene functions at a certain level when we are young and as we age, gene functionality may slow or speed up, leading to a different gene expression profile. The degree of change is related to the rate of aging. (See Chapter 2 for additional information)

LIKE MUSIC TO YOUR EARS (AND YEARS!)

Let me give you an analogy of how balancing Youth Gene Clusters works. When you watch an orchestra, you see and hear how each beautiful sound comes from a particular group. Just as an orchestra plays as a group, genes work in groups to ochestrate cell function. When the orchestra plays in perfect harmony, the result is a perfectly inspiring and beautiful symphony.

Similarly, Youth Gene Clusters work together to harmonize cellular energy, skin appearance, mental clarity, and vitality. With age, these clusters get out of balance; just as an orchestra becomes sharp or flat, and interrupts perfect harmony.

Like any good conductor, ageLOC science identifies and targets the individuals and/or groups that aren't performing up to par. Then, it's simply a matter of retuning the musical instruments and leading the group or individual to play harmoniously once again. With ageLOC science, we're resetting the Youth Gene Clusters to a more balanced and youthful state.

WHEN THE MUSIC STOPS

So, what happens in the 50-year-old body, or the 50-year-old face when it is not balanced with the science of ageLOC? Think of an orchestra in the hands of an amateur. The lack of technical knowledge and conducting makes them not in sync with the musical score as written by the composer. The music coming out of it sounds like when I might try to play Mozart without knowing the score. Similar abuse can occur inside our bodies. The "youth" score is not played correctly. The genes, like strings on a violin, are just not activated correctly. Their expression gets muddled or blurred. They aren't working well together and are not balanced.

TURNING UP THE HEATMAP

We can scientifically "see" how Youth Gene Clusters can be reset to a more youthful balance by looking at a heatmap that shows the expression of various genes. The **heatmap** shown is a graphical representation of gene expression data represented as colors (see color version on page 201). It shows the differences in a whole array of genes with and without the application of ageLOC science. Let me emphasize that it is the activity of genes and not the gene structure that has been changed. None of the genes has been altered structurally.

Can I just say that to me, there is art in science.

AGELOC® YGC HEATMAP

YOUNG GENE EXPRESSION

OLD GENE EXPRESSION

OLD GENE EXPRESSION WITH AGELOC SCIENCE

COLUMN 1

COLUMN 2

COLUMN 3

COLOR RANGE

LOW EXPRESSION

HIGH EXPRESSION

FIGURE DESCRIPTION

This heatmap illustrates gene expression of three groups of mice from a pre-clinical test with ageLOC. Young (column 1), old (column 2), and old with ageLOC science (column 3). Each row represents one of 52 genes comprising the mitochondrial Youth Gene Cluster (mtYGC). Columns 1 and 2 show that each of the 52 genes became more or less active during the aging process. In column 3, the YGC activity pattern of the old with ageLOC science group has been reset to a gene expression pattern more similar to the young group in column 1.

(See full color heat map in the appendix.)

COLUMN 3 SHOWS HOW AGELOC SCIENCE **RESET** GENES TOWARD A MORE YOUTHFUL GENE EXPRESSION PATTERN.

Transcriptional Biomarkers of Mitochondrial Aging and Modulation by Cordyceps Sinensis Cs-4. Gordon Research Conference, Biology of Aging, Determinants of Health-Span: From Cells to Humans, August 22-27, 2010. Les Diablerets Conference Center, Les Diablerets, Switzerland.

See color heatmap on page 205.

Why do cells age? Why don't the genes just tell the cell to stay young?

ANSWER:

There is a constant battle going on between nature and nurture. Genes (nature) are thrown out of whack as the body is bombarded over time by negative environmental factors (nurture). Humans generally take better care of their cars than they do their own bodies. We tend to burn the candle at both ends. We eat a poor diet, live in a poor environment, make poor tobacco and alcohol choices, and sometimes just plain have bad luck.

It's like trying to ride a bicycle forever without cleaning and maintenance. Year after year of use wears it down as its parts get dirty, ground down, gummed up, and worn–out.

Or, think of a vacuum cleaner or a jet engine or anything else mechanical. If they are well maintained, cleaned, and serviced, they can run beautifully (or as we say "youthfully") for a very long time. Without maintenance, they wear out prematurely.

Years ago my computer suddenly crashed. I took it in to be serviced. Now you'll really know how old I am when I tell you that this was in the days when computers used floppy disks. Anyway, the next day when I went to pick it up, the technician handed me a sandwich bag full of pennies, thumbtacks, Cheerios®, buttons, paper clips, and other small little "treasures" my two-year-old had stashed away in the floppy slots.

You see, you just can't put the wrong things into a delicate mechanism (like our bodies) and not have something go screwy! But the body is resilient if given half the chance, and it can and will reset itself when aided properly.

ageLOC can help balance gene expression to behave in a more youthful manner. These marvelous intelligence engines, the genes, are inherently designed to function at their optimal level. They can promote youthful gene expression as long as they are properly influenced.

QUESTION:

How old are you, Joe?

ANSWER:

People stare at me, and I don't blame them. I am the person behind the ageLOC story, and they are curious to know how it's working for me. I can feel their eyes combing my face, looking for any small wrinkles, lines, and age spots. I can tell they are dying to ask me my age, and they're always shocked to find out that I'm actually 58. As you can see from this picture, I look a lot younger.

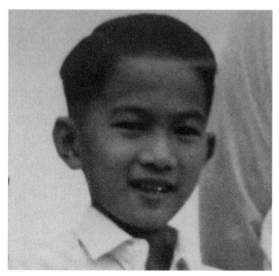

JOSEPH AT 9 YEARS OLD.

Just kidding! ageLOC won't make me 9 again, but it will keep people guessing my real age for years to come!

This might be a good time to show you the real me today.

Okay, ageLOC doesn't guarantee to make you good-looking! But, I can tell you that, in this picture, I feel great. Like a kid again. And people say I look younger than others my own age. My skin looks and feels great. I have energy and vitality to spare.

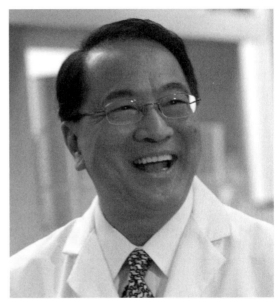

JOSEPH CHANG, PH.D.

QUESTION:

What makes ageLOC unique?

ANSWER:

I believe ageLOC is unique from other technologies out there because of the science. ageLOC technology enables us to decipher and understand the genetic instruction manual. We believe ageLOC gives us important clues about gene expression during aging. We understand how multiple genes work in concert to either accelerate or slow aging. Most importantly, the body is not just a bag of cells; rather, different tissues age differently, depending on their role in the body. ageLOC identifies, targets, and resets these important Youth Gene Clusters to a more youthful pattern.

SURPRISE QUESTION:

I was talking to a couple in Sweden who told me that their daughter was reluctant to use anti-aging products. They were puzzled. They could not imagine why this beautiful 20-year-old girl did not want to maintain her youthful looks and good health. She finally asked, "Am I too young to worry about aging now? Shouldn't I wait until I get old?"

ANSWER:

This is an excellent question. You *do* need to worry about aging *now* because some studies show that the aging process can start early in a very technical and metabolic sense. When you hit your early 20s is typically when you start to worry about your appearance and health. Indeed, in addition to sun exposure, other lifestyle habits can either accelerate or slow aging. While you may not see the immediate impact of lifestyle habits, there is very little doubt that unnoticeable damage accumulates with time. Eventually such damage will be noticeable and before you know it, you are looking old. No matter how young you are, there are some things you should always do to take aging precautions, like using sunscreen, for example.

QUESTION:

Am I actually harming myself by using the wrong products?

ANSWER:

Let me answer this question by posing this scenario. Imagine your frustration waiting for a service call on your clothes dryer and the repairman turns up with the wrong replacement parts for your machine and is confused about exactly what needs maintenance. Your time is wasted, and you still don't have your machine tuned-up and ready to work for you.

That's what happens when products are not carefully evaluated and created with the right science. In order to truly affect aging, we have to understand the fundamental sources of aging and then understand how to influence them effectively. While you may not be "harming" yourself other than wasting time and money, you are certainly not helping yourself.

QUESTION:

Why haven't other companies developed platforms similar to ageLOC science?

ANSWER:

Our knowledge has been accumulated over many years. This ageLOC knowledge, and our expertise, is an unbeatable combination that is both proprietary and patented. When asked if I think our anti-aging science is "better" than our competitors on the market, I humbly reply with a grin, "Yes, better, and SMARTER!"

QUESTION:

Can nutritional supplements really help my genes?

ANSWER:

The body is not just a random bunch of cells; rather, different tissues age differently, depending on their role in the body. Products developed through ageLOC science can reset the relevant Youth Gene Clusters to act younger. This can happen to skin cells to impact the way your skin reflects age with things like lines, wrinkles, and age spots, but the science works exactly the same way inside the body. In your body you have major organs like your liver, kidneys, heart, etc. These organs are made of tissues that are comprised of cells that are communicating in the same delicate balance. When you influence those cells to reflect youthfulness, you get the benefit. This happens through carefully formulated nutritional supplements that incorporate ageLOC science.

QUESTION:

Are nutritional supplements safe?

ANSWER:

Well, let me start this answer by restating what I said earlier in this book; not all products are created equal! When we develop nutritional supplements, we do so with a pharmaceutical-grade manufacturing practice and with substantial research and development going into the science behind the products. This allows me to say with confidence that our nutritional supplements are not only safe, but they are effective. I cannot make that blanket statement for the industry, however, because I don't have influence on the ingredients, manufacturing, and research done on other nutritional supplements out there.

QUESTION:

How do I know if I am already experiencing the signs of aging?

ANSWER:

There are two main concerns with aging: looking older and feeling older. For now, lets focus on *looking* older.

I guarantee that **you are not looking your best (or youngest)** if your skin shows some of the following signs of skin aging:

- FINE LINES AND WRINKLES
- POOR SKIN STRUCTURE
- DISCOLORATION SUCH AS DULL OR SALLOW SKIN, AGE SPOTS, OR DARK EYE CIRCLES
- UNEVEN SKIN TONE OR RUDDY COMPLEXION

- **HYDRATION PROBLEMS SUCH AS DRY, FLAKEY, OR OILY SKIN**
- **POOR TEXTURE**
- **LIFELESS, DULL SKIN**
- **BIG PORES**

If you don't have any of these aging signs, you're probably only six months old. If you do, does it bother you? Would you like to see someone younger staring back at you when you look at yourself in the mirror?

YOUTH GENE CLUSTERS & THE 8 SIGNS OF AGING

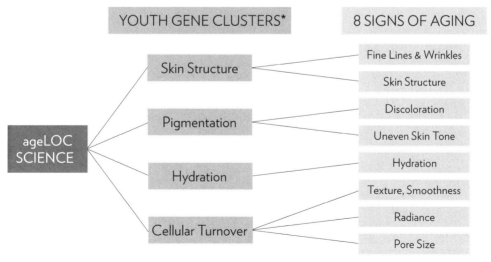

* This is only a selection of meaningful Youth Gene Clusters.

FOUR FOR EIGHT

Our labs have already identified four meaningful and specific functional Youth Gene Clusters that are responsible for these eight aging attributes in the skin. This knowledge guides us in creating products that can improve these key signs of aging.

(See Appendix for more information)

QUESTION:

I recently received the following email: "I am a man in my late sixties. I love the outdoors and have always been an avid sportsman. My face is so brown and wrinkled my wife calls me 'Leather Larry'. Is it too late for me?

P.S. I don't have as much energy as I used to, either. Now THIS I hate."

ANSWER:

No. It's not too late on either count.

It's been said that skin is like an elephant; it never forgets those late nights, stress, pollution, or sunbathing. This is true to some degree. However, I have seen for myself that skin is resilient and when proper care is taken, you have the ability to restore a youthful appearance.

A SECOND CHANCE

ageLOC science may give everyone a second chance at looking and feeling younger without putting the body at risk. ageLOC goes far beyond just concentrating on the *outside* of the body and takes ageLOC *inside*. What good, after all, is health that is only "skin deep?"

If you are interested in the maximum benefits of a **complete youthful revitalization of your body?** *Read on*! I have plenty to say about that in the following chapter.

"I intend to live forever, or die trying!"
GROUCHO MARX

YOU LIVE IN A TIME OF TREMENDOUS TECHNOLOGICAL innovation and advancement. You are among the first generations to have iPods, Internet, smartphones, and the ability to watch any television show anytime, anywhere. You can connect with anyone anywhere in the world while sitting in your home. It's fascinating. Well, just as advances in technology have given you control over so many things from the comfort of your own home, now, science and the understanding of genetics are giving you the opportunity to be the first generation of humans that can actually influence your own aging, again, all from the comfort of your own home! Ponder that fact for a moment. Exciting, isn't it?

ANTI-AGING: THE NEXT TRILLION DOLLAR MARKET

You, and millions of people like you, are hoping and expecting to look and feel as young as possible far into your senior years. I like the term "golden years." Gold is the purest of metals. It has a unique color and shine, which makes it beautiful. It doesn't tarnish. It doesn't corrode. It never loses its integrity under heat or extreme pressure. These are pretty good similes for the elder generation. I think all of us want to "shine" for as long as we live. That's why you and I have such a vested interest in aging well.

Market research proves that anti-aging is a very big deal worldwide. In 2009, a study by BCC Research, "Anti-aging Products and Services: The Global Market," shows that billions of dollars are spent each year for a whole range of anti-aging products and services. Not surprisingly, "baby boomers," those born between 1946 and 1964, comprise 75% of the buyers. Europe is the largest market, followed by the United States and the Asian Pacific area.

An astonishing $162.2 billion was spent in 2008 by boomers and was forecasted to grow at an 11.1% compound annual growth rate. That would bring the total to $274.5 billion by 2013.

People all over the world are clearly willing to make a significant investment into the pursuit of a genuine anti-aging solution. Anti-aging products, once considered "luxury items," have evolved into absolute necessities for millions of people globally. The evidence is clear, people are certainly willing to put their money where their wrinkles are. As I pointed out in previous chapters, they are even willing to go under the knife to try to look young.

WHAT ABOUT YOU

After reading about the benefits of looking and feeling younger, are **you** interested in investing in your health? I truly hope so. Your future depends on how you age, and aging well is a wonderful investment in your future.

CHOOSE WISELY

Before you start investing heavily into your aging future, I want you to be informed. I want you to have all of the facts.

When deciding the products and services that will best support your aging needs, let me remind you that you cannot go deeper into the science of anti-aging research than the genetic level. This is where the meaningful anti-aging solutions will be found.

Remember that products are only as good as the science behind them. You can find plenty of products on the market that will address your immediate needs, but what about the source? If we put a bucket under a leak in our roof, it may catch the water for a while, but what happens when the bucket overflows? We need to fix the leak itself. In other words, go to the source.

When it comes to products, we need to do the same thing. This goes way beyond just producing a good-smelling, herbal hand lotion or face cream to temporarily smooth extra-dry skin, for example. The idea is to understand what is influencing the genes to make better products that actually improve that dry skin condition.

Again, we are trying to truly influence the source of the issue, not just to mask it by addressing only the signs of the real issue.

WHAT'S OUT THERE

The other evening, I stopped by my local bookstore and headed for the magazine section. I wanted to see what was being said about anti-aging. I guess I wasn't too surprised. Nearly every magazine on the rack, women's and men's, had some sort of article on anti-aging. One magazine had literally dozens of advertisements promoting anti-aging products.

A COMPREHENSIVE APPROACH

So, you might wonder just where ageLOC products and innovations fit into this array of magazine promotions I had found. After going through dozens of magazines at the bookstore, I discovered most products did not approach aging at the genetic level, and the ones that did target aging in the genes focused on only one or two genes. As we have discussed in this book, our approach is unique because we focus on clusters of genes to give us a more holistic approach to target aging right at the source.

Of course, this was hardly a valid, scientific survey. It was just me and a lot of magazines spread out on the family room floor. (Side note: I had to try to explain to my wife the sudden interest in women's magazines!) Nevertheless, in all these periodicals, while there were many claims that certain face creams or serums would smooth skin or counteract dryness, there were no references to any products on the market that addressed the underlying causes of aging with a comprehensive genetic-based solution.

AGELOC STANDS ALONE

The reason there is so little available to consumers that addresses the deeper causes of aging skin is that so few companies put the money and time into the science of aging. Do we have ageLOC anti-aging serums, hydrating creams, and antioxidant formulas? Yes, we do. Don't ageLOC products clean, balance, moisturize, tighten, and rejuvenate skin just like the products advertised? Yes, they do. But we provide, I believe, far more for your investment.

Nu Skin, with ageLOC science, stands apart from the competition because our approach is based upon years of anti-aging research. We can identify, target, and reset aging at its source. We have put a "LOC" on our findings and proprietary research and development through comprehensive protection of intellectual property.

With ageLOC's ability to influence the gene expression of aging-related genes, we have created a new paradigm that provides people like you with innovative anti-aging science encompassing both skincare and nutrition. Our exclusive access to information on the sources of aging offers a whole new way of looking at aging. No other company has the technology that identifies multiple aging-related genes and the ability to reset these genes.

AGELOC AS A PLATFORM

By now I hope you're convinced that the old paradigm of "aging is inevitable" needs to be discarded. There is something you can do to influence your inherited genes. With ageLOC's ability to influence the gene expression of aging-related genes, the new paradigm provides an innovative anti-aging platform encompassing both personal care and nutrition. Our exclusive access to information on the sources of aging offers a whole new way of looking at aging. ageLOC has proprietary technology that identifies multiple aging-related genes and how we can begin to reset these genes.

Perhaps this is a good time to discuss with you what ageLOC **is** and what it **is not.**

ageLOC is Nu Skin's entire platform to become the world's leading anti-aging company, including the science, the research, and the methods for unlocking the secret of youth.

We make no false promises here. ageLOC isn't magic. ageLOC will not make us immortal. ageLOC cannot be described as diagnosing, curing, or preventing any disease. Claims like these are drug claims and are in the realm of medicine. ageLOC should not be characterized as gene therapy, genetic engineering, gene-splicing, or any other similar terms. While all these terms relate to specific approaches to influencing genes, Nu Skin's approach is different. It is a holistic and nutritional approach, utilizing ageLOC science to develop products designed to support healthy aging by understanding how to positively influence gene expression.

What ageLOC *is*, is innovative and unlike any other approach to anti-aging. I have not "patented" genes. What we have done is secure over a dozen patents on ageLOC research. This literally locks out competitors from using our proprietary research and development methods and science, which we utilize to develop superior products. With ageLOC, you have come to "the source of the science."

ageLOC is safe. It is about extraordinary measures, not drastic measures. It's about taking yourself on a gentle, sane journey to improving your skin and health as you age. It's about aging beautifully and healthfully. It's about letting your own body rejuvenate itself. It's about owning your youth, and allowing the improvements to come naturally.

Our goal is to extend the qualities of youth into your skin and bodies for as many years as possible.

YOUR GOOD FORTUNE

We live in exciting times, when science gives you remarkable and wonderful control to effect extraordinary change in your life. Take cataracts, for instance.

A cataract is a clouding of the normally clear and transparent lens of the eye. Cataracts can become so opaque and unclear that light cannot easily be transmitted to the retina. In severe cases, this is like a heavily frosted window over someone's ability to see.

I have personally witnessed thousands whose vision is extremely impaired because of cataracts, a condition that medical science can often easily correct, given the right place with the right equipment. Depending on how thick cataracts are, they can be reduced by drugs or they can be removed by surgery. The most recent innovations in cataract surgery involve implanting a new, flexible lens behind the iris of the eye, using a tiny incision that doesn't even need stitches. I've seen this done by my brother-in-law, an opthamalogist who per-forms this surgery as a matter of routine. It's wonderful. In two hours people are walking out of cataract surgery able to see clearly.

So, what does this have to do with you and your anti-aging decisions?

Cataract surgery is a great example of how scientific advancements create modern "miracles" for everyday people. However, it is only available to people who can get it. Sometimes the "miracles" we are looking for are only a matter of access. To those who have access to modern cataract surgery, the technology isn't really miraculous. It is great science and good fortune! But, to those who do not have access, to those who spend their lives in cloudy darkness wishing for something—anything—to take away the fog, getting it would certainly be a "miracle" to them.

YOU HAVE ACCESS

Science has given you the power to manage your own aging destiny. Just like high-tech computers and the Internet have given you the ability to communicate with anyone in the world and find the answers to most questions at the push of a button, science has become the empowering, enabling tool to allow you to do something about aging. ageLOC has given us the explanation and the tool to resolve the problem. And thus you have unlocked the mystery of aging and brought truth to the myths related to aging.

By reading this book, you're one of those fortunate people on earth with access to the science of ageLOC. **You're part of that first generation of people with the knowledge to actually influence the genes that cause aging.** You don't have to take your aging woes to the clinic or the hospital. You have access to the tools to beat the eight signs of aging (fine lines and wrinkles, skin structure, discoloration, uneven skin tone, hydration, texture and smoothness, radiance, and pore size). You don't have to rely on stimulants. You can enhance and influence your vitality without harmful and damaging effects.

You can do all of this as easily as you can wash and moisturize your face or swallow a few capsules.

JUST DO IT

I, my team of research scientists, and the entire Nu Skin organization can, and will, continue to put our best science, efforts, and money into creating the most impressive anti-aging products on the market. Ultimately, however, it is you who will be responsible for discovering how good they really are.

In 1952, Dr. Robert Bruce pioneered the first medical treadmill for the benefit of combating cardiovascular issues and weight gain. Imagine his frustration if he were alive today to see the enormous obesity problem facing the world. The treadmill has been a highly effective tool in the battle against obesity and heart disease—for those who actually utilize this tool. Yet far too many others (millions perhaps) have invested in a treadmill but have it sitting and collecting dust in the corner while their bodies deteriorate and their hearts fail.

I can only imagine how frustrated Dr. Bruce might be today. I feel that same level of anxiety over the realization that my research team and I have unlocked the mysteries of aging and have pioneered real-world solutions, yet far too many people continue to suffer needlessly from the effects of aging.

You have made an investment of time and money into this book which you have now completed. You possess the knowledge and have access to the tools. What's next? Will you place this book on a high shelf and allow it to collect dust with other "good books" you have read in the past, or will you take swift and determined action on your own behalf?

I believe you have already seen some of the effects of aging, be they subtle or significant, which is what drove you to obtain this book. I also believe you are serious about fighting the effects of aging because you have invested enough time reading to arrive here at the final pages of my book. Now comes the most important step in your future aging process—immediate action. I say "immediate" for a couple of reasons.

First of all, studies have shown that if action is not taken immediately after a life-altering decision, the odds of ever taking any action decrease substantially. Your success depends on you moving forward immediately in obtaining the tools to begin your new approach to aging.

The second reason I strongly urge you to take immediate action is because of that grumpy old man known as Father Time. Time is not a friend of aging—quite the contrary, actually. With every passing hour, your cellular structure continues to decline in a number of ways. Every morning millions of people worldwide awaken to look in the mirror and discover a new wrinkle that wasn't there yesterday, or a new symptom of getting older that may have been either prevented or at least postponed had they simply had access to the solutions we have developed with ageLOC.

How many more mornings will you wake up frustrated with that ever-aging reflection in the mirror before you decide to take action? How many more irreversible symptoms of aging can you tolerate before standing up and shouting, "ENOUGH!" I implore you to slam this book shut right now (seriously, slam it shut!) and declare the war against aging *on*!

Join with me and millions of others worldwide in the joyous journey of actually aging with health and youthfulness. Today is your turn!

"In all things of nature there is something of the marvelous."

ARISTOTLE

IT'S QUITE CLEAR BY NOW THAT I AM PASSIONATE ABOUT ageLOC! Why? Because I believe it is the *key* to unlocking a lifetime of answers I have diligently sought in terms of healthy aging. I say key, because ageLOC opens up a promising new science of anti-aging which could prove to be of enormous benefit to you.

Think of it this way. When scientists discovered the key to splitting the atom, thousands of new possibilities in nuclear technology opened up. They didn't invent the atom. They just discovered the key to its enormous possibilities.

It's the same with the advanced research we call ageLOC. We did not invent genes and the marvelous potential locked inside of the genetic code, but vital information encoded in the human genome and recently unlocked has led us to our ageLOC technology.

We, together with our partners, are leading the field with some of the most important anti-aging science undertaken today.

Knowing this, all I can say, in the words of the good-ole-boys is, "This dog will hunt!" We offer you a new playbook with life-altering insight that you can use to play a winning game of anti-aging.

TAKING THE FEAR OUT OF DYING

I sincerely believe that people are not afraid of dying when they have lived a full life. But if they have suffered in their later years and been unable to fulfill their dreams, they come to death with regrets and anxiety.

While some have romanticized the idea of immortality, most people peacefully accept death as a normal, natural transition. What people fear is pain, suffering, disability, and wracking illness. To all of us, such conditions create a frightening end vision of getting old.

I believe some doctors can help their patients with positive, healthy approaches to the ravages of aging.

YOUTHSPAN VS LIFESPAN

ageLOC is about helping people live healthy and productive lives for as long as possible. By adopting the ageLOC approach, you can retain the qualities of youthful life as you age, making later life fulfilling and satisfying.

We live in exciting times. What does this actually mean? "Exciting" brings to mind words like positive, energetic, vibrancy, and on and on. At any level you need healthy living. How can life be exciting if you don't have good health?

Because of the potential of ageLOC, I truly believe that all of us can start referring to our time on this earth as our "youthspan" rather than our lifespan.

We are barely scratching the surface of what we can achieve in terms of aging research. This book explains our incredible breakthroughs and the science behind being able to identify, target, and reset Youth Gene Clusters. And I believe we are only in the early innings of the ageLOC "World Series of Healthy Aging." There are more innings to come.

ageLOC to date has focused on the first three innings: skin **renewal** and **rejuvenation** and protecting the mitochondria as an effective mechanism to **recharge** energy production in the body.

Future innings with ageLOC science may reveal that there are genes responsible for **restoring** the body, and ultimately leading to healthy **regeneration.** How powerfully could this influence how we might **restage** our lives, **rejoicing** in the health we enjoy until the end of life?

TRUST YOUR INSTINCTS

At this juncture, thinking about restaging our lives, we can consider what constitutes a healthy lifestyle. I believe moderation is the formula for healthy aging. Forget about extreme diets, workouts that only a gymnast could do, and loosey, goosey advice from new age "gurus" that defy logic and common sense.

As a human species, we have evolved to a stage where deep within our genetic code we know what is right and what is wrong for our bodies. This instinct can be trusted.

The following summary, based on the universality of common sense and experts around the world, forms the basis of principles that will help you live younger longer.

1. **Decide to be happy.** With this in mind, you will be able to moderate your moods. Laughter and smiling are directly related to better health.

2. **Exercise naturally.** Remember that you come from a hunter-gatherer species. Your body is flexible and mobile. Keep it that way.

3. **Eat a wide spectrum of foods**. Every food has value; it's only the excessive consumption of a particular food that leads to problems. Portion control is the key. Another important idea: Don't eat alone. Think about it. Picture your eating—often snack binging—when you are alone in front of the television, reading a book or surfing the Web.

4. **Bond with people.** Remember, no man is an island. Avoid loneliness by actively joining groups, volunteering and being the one to invite others into your life. Humans are not genetically coded to be hermits.

5. **Rise and shine.** Acclimate your body to the rhythm of the sun.

6. **Read.** I fully believe in the phrase, "A mind is a terrible thing to waste."

7. **Learn to love, forgive, and let things go.** If you let something eat at you, it will consume you.

8. **Manage stress.** Occasional stress that motivates you to action is fine but chronic stress is extremely harmful.

9. **Keep busy.** Another of my favorite phrases, "Idle hands are the devil's workshop," is never more true than today.

NOW YOU ARE UP TO BAT

Earlier I mentioned you are getting a new playbook to use in the game of anti-aging. Let me put some added emphasis on the "you" part of that offer because ultimately, only you can step forward into a far more positive and hopeful aging future.

Your lifespan depends mostly on environment or safety. We all know only too well that a life can be instantly ended because of a natural or unplanned disaster, or a cruel act of someone else's choice.

Your youthspan, however, is all about "how" you age and is far more vulnerable to your own choices. I began this conclusion with a quote from Aristotle. Let me give you another one.

Excellence is never an accident. It is always the result of high intention, sincere effort, and intelligent execution; it represents the wise choice of many alternatives—choice, not chance, determines your destiny.

I would add these four words to the above quote: *"Excellence in YOUR personal health is never an accident."* ageLOC gives you the wherewithal to fuel your high intention to slow the negative effects of biological aging until the very moment you stop aging chronologically. Simply put, ageLOC will give you marvelous tools that, if you choose to employ them, will help you to die healthy.

As Sherlock Holmes is famous for saying, "The game is afoot!" Are you ready to play?

ABOUT THE AUTHOR

"My goal in life has always been to use my interest in science to benefit all people. I believe my work in the underlying causes of aging does just that. It is the ultimate focus on health."

JOSEPH CHANG

JOSEPH CHANG, PH.D., WAS BORN IN IPOH, MALAYSIA, A SMALL community where his great-great grandparents settled after leaving China in the late nineteenth century. His father was a tin miner and his mother a primary school teacher. Joe was especially close to his grandmother, because she was the one who took care of him while his parents worked during the day.

"My grandmother was a traditional Chinese woman who never got more than an elementary education, but she was wise." As he walked to and from school with her, she told him stories of his ancestors, especially his great-grandfather who supported his family tapping latex from rubber trees in the jungle and selling it to the large Malaysian rubber industry.

"What stuck with me over the years was the fact that he began work before dawn, eating only a breakfast of rice gruel and a small piece of vegetable that sustained him throughout the day. Yet, he lived a long life in spite of the difficult work. This impressed and influenced me in my later studies on nutrition and longevity."

It was incredibly important to Joe's parents that their children receive an education. With the unwavering support and sacrifice of his family, Joe and his siblings were the first generation of college-educated members of the Chang family. It was during his early years of education that his keen interest in science emerged.

"My passion from the time I was barely out of my teens was exploring the biological sciences as applied to human health, although I didn't want to be a doctor. Being a doctor alone wouldn't allow me to develop sufficient scientific knowledge to truly study health and disease. I wanted to study the fundamental causes of serious health issues and be a part of discovering solutions."

Joe attended undergraduate school at Portsmouth University in England, married Ping, his high school sweetheart, and went on to earn his Ph.D. in Pharmacology at the University of London in 1978. His research institute was located in the Royal College of Surgeons, one of the oldest surgical colleges in the world. Auspiciously, the college maintains a very impressive and extensive collection of disease tissues. Thus, each day as he went back and forth to classes, Joe would walk past that huge display of dead tissues and wonder, "Why did they have to be that way? Why was disease so prevalent?"

This passion for discovering the essential causes of disease motivated Joe to achieve impressive academic honors including being recruited for a post-doctorate fellowship at Johns Hopkins University School of Public Health and Hygiene in Baltimore, Maryland, USA, where he was named an Arthritis Foundation Fellow. His work there motivated him to focus on health from a preventative viewpoint.

"I was very influenced by the dean of the school, Donald Henderson, who was responsible for leading the effort to eradicate smallpox, a disease which had been the scourge of humankind for centuries. These experiences became powerful influences in my life, driving me to search for answers to human health and what it means to be healthy throughout life."

At both universities, Joe learned that good science involves conducting quality experiments where both positive and negative outcomes are equally valuable.

"It is never just about a single experiment but always learning from each experiment while keeping the overarching scientific mission in mind."

In 1981, Joe began a dynamic career path working for major pharmaceutical companies doing ground-breaking research into a number of critical health issues. He joined important health associations and boards, published ground-breaking books, articles, and reviews on pharmacological research and secured several patents on new drugs. Early in his work at Wyeth-Ayerst Laboratories he learned that the path to developing a drug was both arduous and expensive, requiring an army of scientists and a large budget, all influenced by the monumental task of satisfying the requirements of the U.S. Food and Drug Administration.

He also saw that many new, exciting drug technologies were based on natural products, but because natural ingredients couldn't be patented, pharmaceutical companies were reluctant to invest in them, as there would be no built-in profits that come with exclusive patent rights.

Excited by the treasure trove of health-giving natural products left untapped by the drug industry, he and his friend and colleague, Michael Chang, started a new company, Pharmanex, to focus on developing natural ingredients to maintain and improve health. Pharmanex took both scientists on a journey from the pharmaceutical world to the world of nutritional supplements. Within three years, Pharmanex was sold to Nu Skin which provided the necessary resources for the resulting anti-aging quest that is the mission of ageLOC.

"ageLOC is the fulfillment of my dream to develop the next generation of truly effective anti-aging products."

Today, as Chief Scientific Officer and Executive Vice President of Product Development at Nu Skin Enterprises, Joe passionately works to see his anti-aging vision come to fruition, especially with the advancement of ageLOC technology.

"In all my twenty-five years of research and development of innovative products, ageLOC technology is the most significant in that it holds the greatest potential to help people of all ages! Men and women alike."

Dr. Chang is a member of New York Academy of Sciences, and American Society of Pharmacology and Experimental Therapeutics. He has also served as a Congressional Subcommittee expert witness on marine-derived products. He served on the Board of Directors of a major trade association (CHPA) related to consumer health products in the U.S.

Dr. Chang has published numerous peer-reviewed articles, reviews and books on pharmacological and nutritional research during his 18 years in the healthcare industry, including co-editing a textbook on inflammation, and developing a series of monographs on botanical products to serve as a source of information for consumers and health professionals. Dr. Chang also holds several patents on new drugs in arthritis, asthma, and autoimmune diseases, and is responsible for the discovery of a novel anti-rejection drug called Rapamune® that is derived from natural sources. Rapamune is currently the second-most prescribed drug to prevent organ rejection.

ACKNOWLEDGEMENTS

I AM A MEMBER OF THE VAST COMMUNITY OF SCIENTISTS. This book would not have been possible without the dedication of scientists who have spent their careers on aging research. To these remarkable people, I owe immense gratitude for helping me to understand the aging process through their discoveries. I have approached my study of aging with their help, but I want to emphasize that any errors are my own. Notably, I owe particular thanks to Drs. Tomas Prolla and Richard Weindruch for their outstanding work in the field of genetics and aging. Their pioneering work in nutrigenomics illuminated the road less travelled in aging, and their insights acted as beacons during my quest.

I am also blessed with great scientific colleagues. My heartfelt thanks goes to my stellar R & D team: Mark Bartlett, Helen Knaggs, and all who have contributed to the science of ageLOC. Their intellect and diligence is inspiring and their dedication has made the next generation of anti-aging products a reality.

Nobody understands the struggles and rewards of explaining science to a lay audience better than the Nu Skin marketing team. Special thanks goes to my marketing colleagues, Kevin Fuller, Elizabeth Thibaudeau, Tyler Whitehead, Nate Jackson, and Natalyn Lewis, as well as scientists Angela Mastaloudis and Dale Kern. This entire team lived Hemingway's credo of "grace under pressure;" their collective wisdom made writing this book a joy. No words are enough for this incredible team that managed to translate my scientific jargon into meaningful language.

I am fortunate to work with a world class management team at Nu Skin—Truman Hunt, Ritch Wood, Scott Schwerdt, Matt Dorny, and Dan Chard. Their support of one "mad scientist" has been unwavering. To the founders and the global Nu Skin family, I owe a special debt of gratitude for the opportunity to grow these ideas. My journey with Nu Skin distributors has taught me that it is possible to make a difference every day.

Finally, to my wife, Ping, and my sons, a group hug. I give a special dedication for their support and love along this sometimes-crazy journey. I honor you, and my sincere love and desire is that you may enjoy your years to the fullest.

To each of you who reads the ageLOC story, I say—keep your age a mystery!

JOSEPH CHANG, PH. D., Salt Lake City, Utah.

APPENDIX

CHAPTER ONE

National Institute on Aging (NIA), "An Aging World: 2008."

Kohn, Livia. *Daoism and Chinese Culture.* Three Pines Press. 2001 pp. 4, 84.

Jacobson, Thorkild. *The Sumerian King List.* University of Chicago Press. 1939 pp. 69–77.

Goehlert, Vincent (November 1887). "Statistical Observations upon Biblical Data." *The Old Testament Student.* Chicago: University of Chicago Press 7 (3): 76–83. doi:10.1086/469948.

Li, Mengyu (2008). "The Unique Values of Chinese Traditional Cultural Time Orientation: In Comparison with Western Cultural Time Orientation." The University of Rhode Island.

United Nations (2009). "World Population Ageing." New York, 2010. www.un.org/esa/population/publications WPA2009/WPA2009-report.

Houghton Mifflin Science Education Place.
http://www.HoughtonMifflinEduplace.com.

Comfort, Alex. "The Evolutionary Theory of Aging: Classical
Evolutionary Theories of Aging." http://www.senescience.info.

Hopkin, Karen. "How Long Can People Live?"
http://www.eduplace.com/kids/hmsc/4/a/cricket/ckt_4a3.shtml.

Kinsella, KG. "Changes in Life Expectancy 1900–1990." *AJCN*;
1992;55: 11965–12025. http://www.ajn.org/content/55/6/11965 full.

"Eos and Tithonus." http://www.paleothea.com/Myths/Eos.html.

Moyer, Michael (September 2010). "Eternal Fascinations with the End."
Scientific American, Special Issue—The End. Vol. 303, Num. 3:
Articles: p. 38.

Kirkwood, Thomas (September 2010). "Why Can't We Live Forever?"
Scientific American, Special Issue—The End. Vol. 303, Num. 3:
Articles: p. 42.

CHAPTER TWO

U.S. Department of Energy/National Institutes of Health.
"The Human Genome Project."
http://www.ornl.gov/sci/techresources/Human_Genome/home.shtml.

Venter, Craig, *A Life Decoded: My Genome: My Life.* New York:
Penguin, 2007.

Lee, CK, Weindruch R, Prolla TA. "Gene-expression profile of the ageing brain in mice." *Nat Genet,* 2000;25:294–7.

Lee CK, Klopp RG, Weindruch R, Prolla TA. "Gene expression profile of aging and its retardation by caloric restriction." *Science,* 1999; 285:1390–3.

Park SK, Prolla TA. "Gene expression profiling studies of aging in cardiac and skeletal muscles." *Cardiovasc Res,* 2005; 66:205–12.

Park SK, Kim K, Page GP, Allison DB, Weindruch R, Prolla TA. "Gene expression profiling of aging in multiple mouse strains: Identification of aging biomarkers and impact of dietary antioxidants." *Aging Cell,* 2009; 8:484–95.

Prolla TA. "DNA microarray analysis of the aging brain." *Chem Senses,* 2002; 27:299–306.

Weindruch R. "Caloric restriction, gene expression, and aging." *Alzheimer Dis Assoc Disord,* 2003; 17 *Suppl,* 2:S58–S59.

Weindruch R, Prolla TA. "Gene expression profile of the aging brain." *Arch Neurol,* 2002; 59:1712–4.

Weindruch R, Kayo T, Lee CK, Prolla TA. "Gene expression profiling of aging using DNA microarrays." *Mech Ageing Dev,* 2002; 123:177–93.

Weindruch R, Kayo T, Lee CK, Prolla TA. "Microarray profiling of gene expression in aging and its alteration by caloric restriction in mice." *J Nutr,* 2001; 131:918S–23S.

Anderson RM, Shanmuganayagam D, Weindruch R. "Caloric restriction and aging: studies in mice and monkeys." *Toxicol Pathol*, 2009; 37:47–51.

Ingram DK, Weindruch R, Spangler EL, Freeman JR, Walford RL. "Dietary restriction benefits learning and motor performance of aged mice." *J Gerontol*, 1987; 42:78–81.

Lee CK, Klopp RG, Weindruch R, Prolla TA. "Gene expression profile of aging and its retardation by caloric restriction." *Science*, 1999; 285:1390–3.

Sohal RS, Weindruch R. "Oxidative stress, caloric restriction, and aging." *Science*, 1996; 273:59–63.

Lee CK, Allison DB, Brand J, Weindruch R, Prolla TA. "Transcriptional profiles associated with aging and middle age–onset caloric restriction in mouse hearts." *Proc Natl Acad Sci USA,* 2002; 99:14988–93.

Wanagat J, Allison DB, Weindruch R. "Caloric intake and aging: mechanisms in rodents and a study in nonhuman primates." *Toxicol Sci*, 1999; 52:35–40.

Weindruch R, Walford RL. "Dietary restriction in mice beginning at 1 year of age: effect on life-span and spontaneous cancer incidence." *Science*, 1982; 215:1415–8.

Barger JL, Walford RL, Weindruch R. "The retardation of aging by caloric restriction: its significance in the transgenic era." *Exp Gerontol*, 2003; 38:1343–51.

Park SK, Prolla TA. "Lessons learned from gene expression profile studies of aging and caloric restriction." *Ageing Res Rev*, 2005; 4:55–65.

Ramsey JJ, Harper ME, Weindruch R. "Restriction of energy intake, energy expenditure, and aging." *Free Radic Biol Med*, 2000; 29:946–68.

Colman RJ, Beasley TM, Allison DB, Weindruch R. "Attenuation of sarcopenia by dietary restriction in rhesus monkeys." *J Gerontol*, 2008; 63:556–9.

The American Institute of Biological Sciences. http://www.ActionBioScience.org.

Blue, Laura (February 11, 2010). "Your Kids Could Reach 100." *Time*.

National Human Genome Research Institute, National Institutes of Health (October 2007). "A Guide to Your Genome." *NIH Publication*, No. 07–6284.

Martires K. J., Fu P, Polster AM, Cooper KD, Baron ED. "Factors That Affect Skin Aging: A Cohort-based Survey on Twins." *U.S. National Library of Medicine, National Institutes of Health.* http://www.pubmed.gov.

Guyuron B, Rowe DJ, Weinfeld AB, Eshraghi Y, Fathi A, Iamphongsai S. (April 2009). "Factors contributing to the facial aging of identical twins." *Plast Reconstr Surg*, 123(4):1321–31.

Christensen K, Iachina M, Rexbye H, Tomassini C, Frederiksen H, McGue M, Vaupel JW (March 2004). "Looking old for your age." *Genetics and Mortality. Epidemiology,* 15(2):251–2.

CHAPTER THREE

Associated Press. June 13, 1990.

Chang, J (April 1999). "Scientific evaluation of traditional Chinese medicine under DSHEA: a conundrum. Dietary supplement Health and Education Act." *J Altern Complement Med,* 5(2):181–9.

City Slickers. Directed by Ron Underwood. USA: Castle Rock Entertainment, 1991.

Jack Palance, *youtube.com.*

Ronald Regan, http://www.whitehouse.gov/about/presidents/ronaldreagan. http://articles.cnn.com/2004-06-05/politics/reagan.health_1_ronald-reagan-presidential-library-michael-reagan-maureen-reagan?_s=PM:ALLPOLITICS.

Bob Hope, http://www.bobhope, The official Bob Hope website.

Sheehy, Gail, *Spirit of Survival.* New York: 1987.

Death Becomes Her. Directed by Robert Zemeckis. USA: Universal Pictures, 1992,.

"Aron Ralston Sacrifices His Right Arm to Save His Life." *Carnegie Mellon Magazine.* http://www.cmu.edu/magazine/03fall/aralston.html. "

Ralston, Aron. *Between A Rock And A Hard Place*. New York: Atria, 2005.

http://www.nba.com/history/finals/19971998.html.
http://sports.espn.go.com/espn/espn25/story?page=moments/79.

CHAPTER FOUR

http://www.plasticsurgery.org/x1673.xml?google=risks

Datamonitor: *Weight Management Trends and Behaviors Beyond Dieting and Obesity*, September 2010.

Euromonitor: *Global OTC Healthcare*. "Segmentation and Positioning Create Opportunities in Dietary Supplements," July 2009.

USA Today, Marin Institute, http://thinkdrink.org , http://sciencecases.org, *MNT archives, BBC News, Money Times, AAHPERD Abstracts (March 2010), Guardian, FSA,* and article written by: Catherine Paddock, Ph.D., Copyright: Medical News Today , Not to be reproduced without permission of Medical News Today

http://www.livingsocial.com.

InStyle Magazine; September, 2010, "Beauty: Does it Really Work?" *Marie Claire Magazine*; October, 2010, "Skin Care for Beginners," pp. 266–268.

Daily Health Reviews Newsletter; Dr. Whiting on the Dangers of Energy Drinks; 8/13/2010.

Chang, Joseph, Ph.D. "Perspective: Scientific Evaluation of Traditional Chinese Medicine: Under DSHEA: A Conundrum."

Barrouquere, Brett (September 20). "Caffeine Consumption an Issue in Kentucky Murder Trial." *Associated Press*, Newport, Ky. http://www.5hourenergy.com/ingredients.asp.

Yahoo! Contributor Network (August 28, 2007). "What Are the Dangerous Ingredients in Energy Drinks? The Energy Drink Business Is Booming but All Is not Well for the Consumer." http://www.associatedcontent.com/article/354447/what_are_the_dangerous_ingredients.html?

Teens Doing Botox, with Dr. Bill Johnson. Television Program. CNN, September 7, 2010.

American Society of Plastic Surgeons, 2010 report.

"Side Effects and Dangers of Botox." http://www.essential-botox-resources.com.

Santana, Michelle. "Dangers of Botox." www.ezinearticles.com.

Operation Smile. http://www.operationsmile.org/about_us/contact-us/.

The First Wives Club. Directed by Hugh Wilson. USA: Paramount Pictures, 1996.

Chavis, Jason C. (May 17, 2010). "The World's Deadliest Poison: Botulinum Toxin." http://www.brighthub.com.

Pakhare, Javashree. "Risks and Dangers of Plastic Surgery." http://www.buzzle.com.

Warzak WJ, Evans S, Floress MT, Gross AC, Stoolman S. "Caffeine consumption in children." *The Journal of Pediatrics*, 2010;158(3):508–509.

Seifert SM, Schaechter JL, Hershorin ER, Lipshultz SE. "Health effects of energy drinks on children, adolescents, and young adults." *Journal of the American Academy of Pediatrics*, 2011: 511-528.

CHAPTER FIVE

http://www.seniorjournal.com/NEWS/Features/2007/7-04-13-ActiveRecreation.htm.

Dara Torres, http://www.daratorres.com.

http://www.eldertreks.com.

Harland Sanders, http://www.kfc.com.

Margaret Mead, http://www.mnsu.edu/emuseum/information/biography/klmno/mead_margaret.html.

Grandma Moses, Anna Mary Robertson Moses, http://www.artexpertswebsite.com/pages/artists/moses.php.

Covey, Stephen R. *Seven Habits of Highly Effective People*. New York: Free Press, 1989.

CHAPTER SIX

Morre, D. James, Morre, Dorothy M., (May 17, 2006). "Aging-Related Cell Surface ECTO-NOX Protein, arNOX, a Preventive

Target to Reduce Atherogenic Risk in the Elderly." *Rejuvenation Research*, 9(2): 231–236.; Volume 9: Issue 2: May 17, 2006.

CHAPTER 7

http://articles.latimes.com/2004/feb/16/local/me-bruce16

BCC Research, Market Research Report, "Anti-Aging Products and Services: The Global Market," pp. 4–26, http://www.bccresearch.com, ISBN: 1-59623-479-2.

SUGGESTED READINGS

1. Austad, Steven N. *Why We Age: What Science Is Discovering about the Body's Journey through Life.* New Jersey: Wiley, 1999.

2. Holliday, Robin. *Aging: The Paradox of Life: Why We Age.* New York: Springer, 2010.

3. Kirkwood, Tom. *Time of Our Lives: The Science of Human Aging.* New York: Oxford University Press, 2001.

4. Ridley, Matt. *Genome: The Autobiography of a Species in 23 Chapters.* New York: Harper Perennial, 2006.

5. Stipp, David. *The Youth Pill: Scientists at the Brink of an Anti-Aging Revolution.* New York: Current, 2010.

6. Weindruch, Richard, and Roy L. Walford. *The Retardation of Aging and Disease by Dietary Restriction.* Illinois: Charles C Thomas, 1988.

AGELOC NUTRITION PRESENTATIONS AND PAPERS

Prolla TA. Resveratrol mimics caloric restriction and retards aging in the heart. Oxidants and Antioxidants in Biology, Oxygen Club of California World Congress, March 17–20, 2010, Santa Barbara, CA.

Zhu J, Zhang Y, Yang J, Tan N, Zhao, E Mastaloudis A (presenter). Antioxidation and life span-extension activities of CordyMax in oxidative stress and aging models #A177. Oxidants and Antioxidants in Biology, Oxygen Club of California World Congress, March 17–20, 2010, Santa Barbara, CA. (Received DSM Nutraceutical Research Award)

Tan N, Zhang Y, Yang J, Zhao C, Zhu JS. CordyMax extends the life span in an aging model: a preliminary report, Abstract #A310. Experimental Biology '10, April 24–28, 2010 Anaheim, CA.

Duan L, Zhao C, Liang C, Lu L, Gao L, Li G, Zhu JS. Improvement of exercise metabolism and carotenoid antioxidant scores with CordyMax and LifePak in young Chinese elite athletes, Abstract #D356. Experimental Biology '10, April 24–28, 2010 Anaheim, CA.

Zhu JS, Gao L, Yao Y, Zhou Y. Maturational alteration of differential expressions of GC:AT-biased genotypes of *Cordyceps sinensis* fungi and *Paecilomyces hepiali* in *Cordyceps sinensis*. Abstract #B210. Experimental Biology '10, April 24–28, 2010 Anaheim, CA.

Yang J, Tan N, Zhao C, Zhang Y, Zhu JS. Antioxidation activities of CordyMax in an oxidative stress model: a mechanism of its anti-aging properties. Abstract #311. Experimental Biology '10, April 24–28, 2010 Anaheim, CA.

Barger JL, Mastaloudis A, Prolla TA, Weindruch R, Wood SM,. Provisional Patent on Vitality # 01336-36004, ORAL FORMULATIONS FOR COUNTERACTING EFFECTS OF AGING. Submitted May 24, 2010.

Barger JL, Wood SM, Weindruch R, Prolla TA. Transcriptional biomarkers of age and their modulation by dietary intervention. Colongy, The 1st International Congress on Controversies in Longevity, Health and Aging. Barcelona, Spain, June 24–27, 2010.

Wood SM, Barger JL, Prolla TA, Weindruch R, Mastaloudis A, Ferguson, S. Transcriptional Biomarkers of Mitochondrial Aging and Modulation by *Cordyceps Sinensis* Cs-4. Gordon Conference, Les Diblerets, Switzerland, August 21–27, 2010.

Prolla TA. Mitochondria and Ageing, Japan Symposium. Mechanisms of Ageing and Development 2010; 13:449–450;480–486.

Ferguson SB, Tan N, Dong Y, Lu J, Fisk NA, Wood SM, Zhu JS, Bartlett M. Targeting age-related gene expression improves mental and physical vitality. 1st World Congress on Targeting Mitochondria, Strategies, Innovation and Clinical Applications, Berlin, Germany, November 18–19, 2010.

Wood SM, Ferguson SB, Barger JL, Prolla TA, Weindruch R, Bartlett M. A nutritional strategy to oppose the genetic expression of aging and loss of vitality. 1st World Congress on Targeting Mitochondria, Strategies, Innovation and Clinical Applications, Berlin, Germany, November 18–19, 2010.

Bartlett M. Nutritional and genetic strategies for longevity. Anti-Aging Medical News. Winter 2010:36–40.

Ferguson SB, Tan NZ, Dong YZ, Lu JH, Fisk NA, Wood SM, Zhu JS, Bartlett M. Targeting age-related gene expression improves mental and physical vitality. 1st World Congress on Targeting Mitochondria, Strategies, Innovations & Clinical Applications, November 18-19, 2010, Berlin, Germany.

Li CL, Nicodemus KJ, Baker C, Hagan RD, Chang J, Zhu JS. CordyMax improves aerobic, cardiovascular, and metabolic capacity during exercise in endurance-conditioned athletes. 2002. November 28, 2005.

Wood SM, Barger JL, Prolla TA, Weindruch R, Mastaloudis A, Ferguson SB. Transcriptional biomarkers of mitochondrial aging and modulation by Cordyceps sinesis CS-4. Biology of Aging, Determinants of Health-Span: From Cells to Humans, Gordon Research Conferences, August 22–27, 2010, Les Diablerets, Switzerland.

Wood SM, Ferguson SB, Barger JL, Prolla TA, Weindruch R, Bartlett M. A nutritional strategy to oppose the genetic expression of aging and loss of vitality. 1st World Congress on Targeting Mitochondria, Strategies, Innovations & Clinical Applications, November 18–19, 2010, Berlin, Germany.

Zhao CS, Yin WT, Wang JY, Zhang Y, Yu H, Cooper R, Smidt C, Zhu JS. CordyMax Cs-4 improves glucose metabolism and increases insulin sensitivity in normal rats. J Altern Complement Med. 2002 Jun; 8(3):309–14.

Zhu JS, Halpern GM, Jones K. The scientific discovery of an ancient Chinese herbal medicine: Cordyceps sinesis. Part I. J Altern Complement Med 4(3); 1998:289–303.

Zhu JS, Nicodemus KJ, Hagan RD, Baker C. CordyMax Cs-4 improves cardiovascular and metabolic capacity during exercise in highly fit athletes. FASEB J 2002; (abstr).

Zhu JS, Zhang Y, Yang JY, Tan N, Zhao C, Mastaloudis A. Antioxidation and life span extension activities of Cordyceps sinesis CS-4 in oxidative stress and aging models. Oxygen Club of California World Congress, March 17–20, 2010, Santa Barbara, CA.

Kim SK. Common aging pathways in worms, flies, mice and humans. J Exp Biol 2007; 210(PT 9):1607–12.

Rodwell GE, Sonu R, Zahn JM, Lund J, Wilhelmy J, Wang L, Xiao W, Mindrinos M, Crane E, Segal E, Myers BD, Brooks JD, Davis RW, Higgins J, Owen AB, Kim SK. A transcriptional profile of aging in the human kidney. Plos Biol 2004; 2(12):E427.

Zahn JM, Kim SK. Systems biology of aging in four species. Curr Opin Biotechnol 2007; 18(4):355–9.

Zahn JM, Sonu R, Vogel H, Crane E, Mazan-Mamczarz K, Rabkin R, Davis RW, Becker KG, Owen AB, Kim SK. Transcriptional profiling of aging in human muscle reveals a common aging signature. Plos Genet 2006; 2(7):E115.

Morré DM, Morré DJ, Meadows C, Draelos Z, and Kern, DG. Age-Related Oxidase (arNOX) Implicated in "Aging-Related Oxidative Damage to Skin Proteins." Presented at Oxygen Club of California, 2010 World Congress, Santa Barbara, California, March 2010.

Knaggs H. "Aging and Genes—the Link with Skin," presented at New York Society of Cosmetic Chemists Meeting, March 2010.

Gopaul R and Knaggs H. Regulating the Expression of Genes Associated with the Synthesis and Maintenance of Dermal Hyaluronan and Barrier Lipids Via Topical Treatment of Salicin—An In Vitro Analysis, Society for Investigative Dermatology; J. Invest Dermatol 130. S. 84, May 2010.

Gopaul R and Knaggs H. Salicin Reduces the Expression of Genes Associated with Skin Inflammation—An In Vitro Analysis, Society for Investigative Dermatology; J. Invest Dermatol 130. S. 85, May 2010.

Morré DM, Morré DJ, Meadows C, Draelos Z, and Kern DG. "Inhibition by Coenzyme Q10 of Age Related Oxidase (arNOX) Caused Oxidative Damage in Skin Proteins." Presented at International Coenzyme Q Association Meeting, Brussels, Belgium, May 2010.

Knaggs H. Impact of Scientific Innovations on the Personal Care Industry, *Journal of Cosmetic Science*, 9(3) 2010; 260–263.

Gopaul R, Gibson M, Knaggs H, Holley KC, and Lephart J. An Evaluation of the Effect of a Topical Product Containing Salicin on the Visible Signs of Human Skin Aging, *Journal of Cosmetic Dermatology*, 9(3) 2010: 196–201.

Morré DJ, Morré DM, Kern DG, Wood SM, Toyoda H, and Knaggs H. "Appearance in Japanese Women Correlates with the Presence of Inosotides and Lysolipids, Both Significant Inhibitors of Age-Related NADH Oxidase Levels". Presented at 40th Annual European Society For Dermatological Research, September 2010.

Kern DG, Meadows C, Fuller BB, Knaggs H, Morré DM, and Morré DJ. "Anti-Aging Effects of Superoxide Reduction in Skin by the Application of Specific Inhibitors of Age-Related NADH Oxidase (arNOX)". Presented at International Federation of Societies of Cosmetic Chemists, Buenos Aires, Argentina, September 2010.

Gopaul R, Langerveld A, Knaggs H, and Lephart J. Salicin. "Regulates the Expression of 'Functional Youth Gene Clusters' to Reflect a More Youthful Skin Profile." Presented at International Federation of Societies of Cosmetic Chemists Annual Meeting, Buenos Aires, Argentina, September 2010.

Knaggs H. "Genes and Aging: Links to Skin." Presented at Cosmetics Asia, Bangkok, Thailand, November 2010.

Knaggs H. "Why Do People Look Younger for Their Age," Presented at Asian Cosmetic Chemistry Society, Singapore, China, November 2010.

Gopaul R. "A Review of Current Genomic Techniques Used in Gene Expression Profiling of the Skin." Presented at Society of Cosmetic Chemists Annual Meeting, New York, New York, December 2010.

Gopaul R, Langerveld A, Lephart J, Knaggs HE. New skin benefits identified for white willow bark extract.Society of Cosmetic Chemists Technology Showcase 2009.

Kern D, Morré DM, Morré DJ, Draelos Z. Controlling reactive oxygen species at their source to reduce skin aging. Rejuvenation Research 2010.

Knaggs HE. A new source of aging. J Cosmet Dermatol 2009; 8(2):77–82.

Knaggs HE. The ARNOX enzyme. Cosmetics and Toiletries 2009; 124:48–52.

Morré DM, Meadows C, Hostetler B, Weston N, Kern D, Draelos Z, Morré DJ. Age related ENOX protein ARNOX activity correlated with oxidative skin damage in the elderly. Biofactors 2009; 34(3):237–44.

Morré DM, Morré DJ, Rehmus W, Kern D. Supplementation with CoQ10 lowers age-related (AR) NOX levels in healthy subjects. Biofactors 2008; 32(1–4):221–30.

NU SKIN ENTERPRISES ANTI-AGING SCIENTIFIC ADVISORY BOARD

DAVID J. BEARSS, PH.D.

Co-director, Center for Investigational Therapeutics, Huntsman Cancer Institute, Salt Lake City, Utah. Associate Professor, Department of Oncological Sciences, University of Utah School of Medicine

Dr. Bearss is an expert in small-molecule drug development and in the use of genetic model systems in drug discovery. He has extensive experience in translational research focused on drug development and the use of genetic markers to predict drug sensitivity. As an expert in the regulation of gene expression and genetic model systems, Dr. Bearss brings more than 15 years of genetics experience to Nu Skin's Anti-Aging Scientific Advisory Board. He has published more than 50 manuscripts and book chapters, has more than 20 patents issued or pending, and has received several awards for his scientific achievements. Dr. Bearss was a faculty member at the University of Arizona from 1999-2003 and then founded Montigen Pharmaceuticals where he served as chief scientific officer until Montigen was acquired by SuperGen in 2006. He also held the post of chief scientific officer at SuperGen, overseeing early drug discovery and development. Dr. Bearss received a bachelor's degree in Human Biology from Brigham Young University and earned a doctorate in Cellular and Structural Biology from the University of Texas Health Sciences Center.

LARS BOHLIN, PH.D.

Professor of Pharmacognosy, University Of Uppsala, Sweden

For more than 30 years, Dr. Bohlin has been dedicated to studying, researching, and teaching in the field of pharmacognosy. He earned his M.S. degree in Pharmacy at the Royal Institute of pharmacy in Stockholm in 1972. Then in 1978, he earned his Ph.D. in Pharmacognosy at the University of Uppsala. After his post-doctoral training, together with Professors Carl Djerassi and Paul J. Scheuer, USA, Dr. Bohlin developed marine pharmacognosy in Sweden with the aim to identify structure-activity relationships with potential in drug discovery. He is widely consulted as an expert by both private and public organizations, such as several research councils in Europe. He is subject editor for *Phytochemistry Letters* and a member of the editorial advisory board of *Journal of Natural Products, Planta Medica,* and *Phytomedicine.* He has co-authored more than 130 research articles, reviews, and book chapters. In 2010, he co-authored the sixth edition of the pharmacognosy textbook, *Drugs of Natural Origin—A Treatise of Pharmacognosy.* Dr. Bohlin is also involved in several patent applications and commercial development of bioactive natural products.

MICHAEL N. CHANG, PH.D.

Pharmaceutical Science Advisor

Dr. Chang received a Ph.D. and M.S in Organic Chemistry from Brandeis University and postdoctoral from MIT. As a scientific advisor to Nu Skin, Dr. Chang is an expert in supplement development. He served as the CEO and president of Optimer Pharmaceuticals, Vice President of Research and Development for Pharmanex, the Director of Medical Chemistry at Rhone-Poulenc Rorer, and Deputy Director of Medicinal Chemistry at Merck. He has more than 20 years of pharmaceutical experience, and his previous management responsibilities include the direction of several drug discovery projects and IND submissions. His research has resulted in 35 patents and has been the topic of more than 60 articles published in peer-review journals.

PAUL ALAN COX, PH.D.

Director of the Institute for Ethnomedicine

One of the world's top ethnobotanists, Dr. Cox specializes in the use of plants by indigenous cultures. During his career, he has published more than 150 scientific articles and three books. Dr. Cox received his M.Sc. in ecology at the University of Wales as a Fullbright Fellow. In 1978, Dr. Cox entered Harvard as a Danforth Fellow and National Science Foundation Fellow, and in 1981 he received his Ph.D. in biology. He was later awarded a National Science Foundation Presidential Young Investigator Award by President Ronald Reagan. Currently, Dr. Cox serves as Chairman of the Seacology Foundation, an organization he founded to assist in preserving island rain forests and cultures.

CARL DJERASSI, PH.D.

Emeritus Professor of Chemistry, Stanford University

Carl Djerassi is one of the few American scientists to have been awarded both the National Medal of Science (for his work on the birth control pill) and the National Medal of Technology (for promoting new approaches to insect control). Dr. Djerassi earned his Ph.D. at the University of Wisconsin–Madison, in 1945. A member of the U.S. National Academy of Sciences and the American Academy of Arts and Sciences as well as many foreign academies, Djerassi has received 21 honorary doctorates together with numerous other honors, including the first Wolf Prize in Chemistry, the first Award for the Industrial Application of Science from the National Academy of Sciences, the Erasmus Medal of the Academia Europeae, the Perkin Medal of the Society for Chemical Industry, the Gold Medal of the American Institute of Chemists, and the American Chemical Society's highest award, the Priestley Medal.

ZOE DIANE DRAELOS M.D., F.A.A.D.

Dermatologist and Editor-In-Chief, *Journal of Cosmetic Dermatology*

Dr. Draelos is a practicing, board-certified dermatologist and a Fellow of the American Academy of Dermatology with a research interest in cosmetics, toiletries, and biologically active skin medications. She is a consulting professor in the Department of Dermatology at Duke University School of Medicine and has a clinical practice in High Point, North Carolina. She has been a visiting professor at more than 45 medical institutions nationally and internationally. She is the author of nine textbooks, including *Cosmetics in Dermatology*. Dr. Draelos has contributed chapters to 23 textbooks, written 300 published papers, and currently serves on eight journal editorial boards. In 2006, she received a cosmetics industry lifetime achievement award from Health Beauty America for her research contributions in topical formulations.

GEORGES M. HALPERN, M.D., PH.D.

Professor of Pharmaceutical Sciences, Hong Kong Polytechnic University

Dr. Halpern practiced internal medicine, allergy, and immunology in Paris (1964–1987) and conducted research in allergy, immunology, psychopharmacology, nutrition, and public health. Since 1964, Dr. Halpern has lectured in more than 79 countries, specializing in allergy and control of environment, immunology, infectious diseases, nutrition, health benefits of wine, psychopharmacology, psychosocial interactions, and many other fields related to healthcare. After running a seminar for the Chinese Academy of Sciences in November 2002, he was offered a Distinguished Professorship by the Hong Kong Polytechnic University, Department of Applied Biology and Chemical Technology. He currently serves in the directorate of the State Key Laboratory of Modern Chinese Medicine and Molecular Pharmacology in Shenzhen, China.

STUART K. KIM, M.D.

Professor of Developmental Biology and Genetics, Stanford University

Stuart K. Kim, Ph.D., is a professor of Developmental Biology and Genetics at Stanford University School of Medicine, as well as a faculty affiliate to the Stanford Center on Longevity. As a researcher he has developed DNA microarrays for C. elegans and used them to profile gene expression during development and aging. He has also assembled large data sets from microarray experiments and used them to find sets of co-regulated genes acting as genetic modules.

Dr. Kim has been a Markey Scholar and a Searle Scholar. He is currently an Ellison Scholar for his research on the genetics of aging. He was awarded the Ho-Am Prize in medicine in 2004 and is an editor of *PLOS Genetics*. He is on the National Science Advisory Council for the American Federation for Aging Research and the Scientific Advisory Board of the Buck Institute for Age Research.

ALEXA BOER KIMBALL M.D., M.P.H.

Associate Professor, Harvard Medical School Vice Chair,
Department of Dermatology, Massachusetts General Hospital

Dr. Kimball received her medical degree from Yale University School of Medicine and her masters of public health degree from Johns Hopkins School of Public Health. Dr. Kimball's work includes studies of therapies for disorders such as psoriasis, atopic dermatitis, acne, and superficial basal cell carcinoma. She has presented her work at national and international medical and scientific symposia and has contributed significantly to medical literature. Her articles and abstracts have been published in such journals as *Archives of Dermatology* and *Journal of the American Academy of Dermatology*, and her book chapters have appeared in several editions of eMedicine Dermatology. Highly involved in the medical community, Dr. Kimball currently serves as Director of the Clinical Unit for Research Trials in Skin.

(CURTIS) MAKOTO KURO-O, M.D., PH.D.

Associate Professor of Pathology, University of Texas Southwestern Medical Center

Dr. Kuro-o received an M.D. in 1985 from the University of Tokyo, Japan. He completed his residency training at Tokyo Metropolitan Geriatric Hospital in 1988, after which he returned to the University of

Tokyo as a clinical fellow in cardiology until 1998. He received a Ph.D. in 1991 from the University of Tokyo, following which he pursued postdoctoral training at the National Institute of Neuroscience in Japan. During his postdoctoral work, he identified the klotho gene—an aging suppressor gene in mammals. In 1998, he became an Assistant Professor of Pathology at the University of Texas Southwestern Medical Center at Dallas. His laboratory focuses on understanding the molecular mechanism by which the klotho protein suppresses aging.

LESTER A. MITSCHER, PH.D.

Professor, Department of Medicinal Chemistry, University of Kansas

Dr. Mitscher received his Ph.D. in Chemistry in 1958 from Wayne State University, Detroit, where he studied natural product chemistry. In 1975, he accepted a University Distinguished Professorship and Chairmanship in the Department of Medicinal Chemistry at the University of Kansas. He returned to the faculty in 1992, where his current research includes antibiotics, genetics, and chemoprevention. He has published more than 280 research papers, authored and coauthored seven books on drug discovery, serves on the editorial board of several technical journals, and holds 15 U.S. and global patents. He is a member of the executive committee of the International Organization for Chemistry in Developing Countries and the Senior Advisory Committee of the Global Alliance for TB Drug Development.

KOJI NAKANISHI, PH.D.

Centennial Professor of Chemistry, Columbia University

The very first research on ginkgo biloba, 30 years ago, was the work of Dr. Nakanishi, who isolated the active component of ginkgo.

During his highly productive career, he has advanced the understanding of natural products by determining the chemical structure of nearly 200 bioactive compounds and how they function to affect human, plant, and animal life. He has been given awards by nearly a dozen nations and numerous scientific organizations. He has published 700 scientific papers and written nine books, including an autobiography, *A Wandering Natural Products Scientist* (1991). He is also a recipient of the prestigious King Faisal International Award in the area of science.

LESTER PACKER, PH.D.

Adjunct Professor, Department of Pharmacology and Pharmaceutical Sciences, School of Pharmacy, University of Southern California Distinguished Professor, Chinese Academy of Sciences, Institute of Nutritional Sciences, Shanghai, China

Regarded as the world's foremost antioxidant research scientist, Dr. Packer received his Ph.D. in Microbiology and Biochemistry from Yale University and served as a Professor and Senior Researcher at the University of California at Berkeley for 40 years. Most recently, Dr. Packer has established a research laboratory in the Department of Molecular Pharmacology at the University of Southern California to pursue studies related to the molecular, cellular, and physiological aspects of free radical and antioxidant metabolisms in biological systems. Dr. Packer is the recipient of numerous scientific achievement awards and serves on editorial advisory boards for scientific journals related to biochemistry, antioxidant metabolism, and nutrition. Dr. Packer has published over 700 scientific papers and 70 books on every aspect of antioxidants and health, including *The Antioxidant Miracle*.

TOMAS A. PROLLA, PH.D.

Co-Founder, LifeGen Technologies Professor,
Departments of Genetics and Medical Genetics, University of Wisconsin

Tomas A. Prolla, Ph.D., studied in the Department of Molecular Biophysics and Biochemistry at Yale University, receiving a doctoral degree in 1994. He completed postdoctoral training at the Human and Molecular Genetics Department at Baylor College of Medicine then joined the faculty of the Department of Genetics and Medical Genetics at the University of Wisconsin in 1997. Dr. Prolla has received several awards of scientific excellence, including the Shorb Lecturer Award, the Burroughs Wellcome Young Investigator Award, the Basil O'Connor Starter Scholar Research Award, and the Howard Hughes Medical Institute New Faculty Startup Award. Dr. Prolla's work currently focuses on the use of gene expression profiling, lifespan studies, and histopathology. In 2001, he and Dr. Richard Weindruch founded LifeGen Technologies, LLC—a company focused on nutritional genomics, including the impact of nutrients and caloric restriction on the aging process. Dr. Prolla has published several articles in prestigious scientific journals such as *Science*.

HILDEBERT WAGNER, PH.D.

Professor Emeritus, Institute of Pharmacy, Ludwig-Maximilians University
Center for Pharmaceutical Research, Munich, Germany

Author of *Immunmodulatory Agents from Plants* (Birkhauser Verlag, Basel, 1999), Dr. Hildebert Wagner has studied pharmacy since 1950. He has authored seven other books and more than 900 scientific publications. Dr. Wagner was made a Full Professor of Pharmacognosy in 1965 and later served as Director of the Institute of

Pharmaceutical Biology in Munich until 1999. He has been distinguished by many international scientific institutions including the Universities of Ohio, Budapest, and Debrecen, Dijon, and Helsinki for his work in pharmacy. Dr. Wagner sits on advisory and editorial boards for *Phytochemistry, The Journal of Ethnopharmacology,* the *Journal of Natural Products,* as well as serving as editor for the *International Journal of Phytomedicine.*

DR. RICHARD WEINDRUCH, PH.D.

Co-Founder, LifeGen Technologies, Professor of Geriatrics and Gerontology, University of Wisconsin Department of Medicine

Dr. Weindruch earned his Ph.D. in Experimental Pathology at UCLA in 1978. He is the author and co-author of more than 170 publications, and his scientific awards include the Harman Research Award, American Aging Association (2000) and the Glenn Award, GSA (2000). Dr. Weindruch's research career has focused on the biology of aging and age-related diseases, studying caloric restriction, which slows the aging process and retards the appearance of a broad spectrum of diseases in diverse animal populations. In 2001, he and Dr. Tomas Prolla founded LifeGen Technologies, LLC—a company focused on nutritional genomics, including the impact of nutrients and caloric restriction on the aging process. Dr. Weindruch has published several articles in *Science* and other prestigious scientific journals.

6A Advantage:

Nu Skin is centered on 6 attributes that give the company its competitive advantage:

1. **Aging Gene Databank:** Exclusive access to a proprietary databank containing comprehensive nutrition, youthful, aging, and CR gene expression data.

2. **Assets:** Nu Skin's 16 patents to protect its unique anti-aging products.

3. **Academic All-Stars:** Experienced scientists on our Scientific Advisory Board and our partnerships with LifeGen Technologies and Stanford University.

4. **ageLOC Algorithm:** Proprietary methodology for developing anti-aging products through genetic research allowing us to identify, target, and reset Youth Gene Clusters to target the ultimate sources of aging.

5. **ARMs, or Aging Response Modulators:** Products that allow us to reset Youth Gene Clusters to promote a more youthful pattern of activity.

6. **Array of Expertise:** A global team of Nu Skin and Pharmanex scientists from diverse—yet complementary—disciplines to bring you the most innovative technologies in order to dominate the anti-aging industry.

ageLOC:

Nu Skin's unique anti-aging platform that provides a transformative approach to anti-aging by targeting aging at its source through proprietary ageLOC science in skin care and nutrition.

ageLOC Science:

Developed by Nu Skin in collaboration with leading scientists, ageLOC science identifies and targets the internal sources of aging that contribute to how we look and feel as we age. Nu Skin calls these sources age-related supermarkers, or arSuperMarkers. Once identified, Nu Skin's exclusive ageLOC science targets these arSuperMarkers—the ultimate sources of aging that can influence how we age.

Aging Response Modulators (ARMs):

A new class of anti-aging products that target functional Youth Gene Clusters (YGCs), or similar age-related supermarkers (arSuper-Markers) that influence the aging process, resetting them to a more youthful activity pattern. ARMs cover both skin care and nutritional product categories.

ATP (adenosine triphosphate):

ATP is a nucleotide derived from adenosine; the major source of energy for cellular reactions. ATP serves as the primary source of energy for most physiological and metabolic reactions in the body. As such, ATP is frequently referred to as "cellular energy."

Biological Age:

Age determined by physiology (including how you look and feel). Factors for measuring biological age include changes in the physical structure of the body as well as changes in its performance due to genetics and other factors. Biological age may improve or deteriorate based on health, diet, environment, and other lifestyle factors.

Caloric Restriction (CR):

The only intervention proven to extend healthy lifespan (slow the aging process) and increase maximum lifespan in a variety of species from fruit flies to dogs to primates. CR involves a 30–40% reduction in caloric intake compared to average intakes. CR restricts macronutrient intake (calories in the form of carbohydrates, fats and proteins) with all of the important vitamins and minerals restored through supplementation and/or dietary fortification. Scientists have demonstrated that CR dramatically slows the aging process and is, therefore, a very good model for studying aging and aging interventions.

Chronological Age:

Age measured by amount of time (years and months) that an individual has lived.

DNA (Deoxyribonucleic acid):

The genetic material found in nearly every cell of the human body. DNA contains the genetic information necessary for building and maintaining an organism. Human DNA exists as a double strand known as a double helix, which is tightly bound to form a structure known as a chromosome.

Gene Expression:

The production of a gene product (a protein or a functional RNA). The way in which genes communicate with the cell.

Genes:

The basic units of heredity in living organisms, genes are functional units of DNA. Genes hold the information to build, maintain, and regenerate cells and pass genetic traits to offspring. Some of these traits are fixed, such as eye color or number of limbs, while others change in expression over time, influencing the rate of aging, health and susceptibility to disease. Gene products are predominantly functional proteins that regulate cellular activity.

Genetics:

The study of genes, heredity, and variation in living organisms.

Heatmap:

Data visualization that uses color to represent numbers in a two-dimensional image.

Mitochondria:

The double-membrane, energy-producing, subcellular structure in which aerobic metabolic reactions occur, including fatty acid oxidation and oxidative phosphorylation. Often referred to as the "power houses" of the cell, mitochondria are responsible for the majority of ATP production in the cell. These are the organelles that supply most of the cellular energy in the form of ATP. Mitochondria also appear to be involved in the aging process.

Resetting Youth Gene Clusters:

A phrase that Nu Skin uses to define modulating Youth Gene Cluster expression at levels characteristic of a more youthful state.

Ultimate Sources of Aging:

A phrase that Nu Skin uses to define components of cellular functions and controls that are at the core of why and how we age— what Nu Skin calls age-related supermarkers or arSuperMarkers.

Youth Gene Clusters:

A term that Nu Skin uses to define functional groups of genes whose coordinated expression may be associated with a more youthful state. ageLOC science identifies and resets Youth Gene Clusters to provide benefits in preserving a more youthful state and in reducing the signs of aging. Youth Gene Clusters are a key arSuperMarker. Although Youth Gene Clusters are associated with a specific aging attribute, they are not necessarily located near each other in the genome. Additionally, they may or may not reside on the same chromosome or be a part of the same metabolic pathway.

AGELOC EXPERIENCES

The following are a few selected testimonials about ageLOC science.

My experience with ageLOC Vitality has been great! I feel that I am able to accomplish more each day at work and at home. And after a long day at work, I'm able to stay awake and alert enough to enjoy time with my family. I love my newfound life!

KIM C., Provo, UT

I was a little apprehensive as to what ageLOC Vitality would do or how I would feel after using it. By the second week, I really saw improvement in my overall energy, and a significant improvement in my workouts. I've never taken another product that provides this type of a sustained, healthy lift for me.

SCOTT B., Santa Barbara, CA

Personally, I have never felt better than I feel right now. With ageLOC Vitality, I have increased mental clarity, muscle stamina, and just a feeling of general youthfulness. I feel like a teenager.

SCOTT S., Provo, UT

I am so blessed to use ageLOC Vitality. I feel excited to wake up and start my day and feel like I want to start projects.

CLAUDIA B., Playa del Rey, CA

I just started taking ageLOC Vitality last month and I am so excited about how it has changed my life. It used to be hard for me to get up and work out in the mornings, and now I have the energy to go to the gym and workout longer. What's more, the energy lasts all day and I don't get the midday crash like I used to. I've also noticed that I have increased concentration throughout the day.

RYAN M., Provo, UT

ageLOC Vitality has really changed my life. As a student, I used to struggle with keeping my concentration in all my classes every day. My friend that I play basketball with on the weekend recommended ageLOC Vitality as a way to increase my concentration and energy. I have been taking Vitality for three weeks and I can already see a major difference. I have more energy throughout the day and still have the mental clarity I need to study at night. The increased energy and stamina have also helped me improve my game. My buddy jokes that he regrets telling me about Vitality now!

JOSEPH J., Provo, UT

In 2010, I was doing some P.R. work for the Sundance Film Festival in Park City. Because I had to attend a party one evening, I went to get a manicure and pedicure. A woman next to me was talking on and on about this amazing skincare product and when I saw her face, I asked what she was doing to look so young. Four hours later, I was in her sister's home, getting a half-face facial with the ageLOC Galvanic Spa and Transformation gels. I love what it did for my skin. Now I use all of the ageLOC products I can get my hands on faithfully, including Vitality, and I look and feel absolutely great!

JILL W., Thousand Oaks, CA, Nu Skin Distributor

As a pharmaceutical rep, I always had to look like Barbie. I started down the road of procedure after procedure at 39, but I started to think I had to find a better way, and I did with Nu Skin and ageLOC. In just 90 days, I looked three years younger. Now I'm a Nu Skin junkie.

COLLEEN H., Boise, ID, Nu Skin Distributor

I've been using ageLOC Transformation for ten months and am so pleased with the results! For years, I have had a problem with skin discoloration as a result of taking birth control pills when I was younger. I have always heard that skin discoloration "face masks" can become worse during pregnancy but now, in my seventh month of pregnancy, I am happy to report that the discoloration has actually continued to fade. Since I started using ageLOC, my friends and family have all commented on how radiant and smooth my skin is. I'm definitely hooked!

ERIN P., Pleasant Grove, UT, Nu Skin Employee

KEEP YOUR AGE A MYSTERY CONTESTANTS

I chose to participate in the Keep Your Age a Mystery contest to demonstrate how ageLOC has had profound benefits in my life. ageloc emphasizes change for the good on a deeper level. It is an excellent product that exemplifies the statement "beauty from within," targeting aging at its source and not just on a superficial level.

ETHEL AND APRIL

Never in my 58 years have I encountered such amazing products that have given me such glow and radiance and have diminished my fine lines and wrinkles as ageLOC has. I've used ageLOC products ever since I joined Nuskin (the ageLOC gels in particular) and can feel the smoothness of my skin. I've also started using ageLOC Transformation and am confident that with continued use, the look and feel of my skin will improve significantly and my skin discoloration and pore size will be greatly reduced.

HAYDEE AND JANZ

I am Italian, and in my culture, looking good and taking care of our image is a must! ageLOC has made it easier for me to look great and younger!

MASSIMILIANO AND ALEXIS

ageLOC is my trusted friend that is with me every day, morning and night! In fact, the morning of this photo, I used 20 Nu Skin products. I started with ageLOC Gentle Cleanse & Tone, "Galvanized," used my ageLOC skincare products and Nu Skin makeup, and took LifePak Nano and a shot of g3 as I walked out the door! That evening, my LifePak Nano and ageLOC Future Serum were waiting for me! ageLOC keeps me looking young and I can't wait to add ageLOC Vitality to my daily regimen to help me feel young, too!

RICHELLE AND JENNIFER

I thought my years as a tennis coach in the scorching hot sun had dampened my dream of having good skin. Then I discovered ageLOC and have never been so sure about winning the anti-aging battle until I saw the remarkable transformation on my skin! My pores are finer, dark spots have significantly reduced, and most importantly, my facial contours are tighter than ever.

SAM AND PAULINE

ageLOC products are so simple to use and give me a radiant, fresh, and youthful look. ageLOC gives me a sense of confidence in knowing that my skin is looking the best that it possibly can and I love how it has become difficult for people to guess my age. Because of the effectiveness of these products, I am able to easily share my success story with others. I am grateful to Nu Skin for providing us with an extremely competitive product that will surely improve the lives of others who use it.

TERRI AND DOMINIQUE

I have been getting lots of compliments from friends on how much younger I look compared to even just 3 months ago! My kids are now often mistaken as my siblings or friends!

AMY AND GABRIEL

My mother and I have been using Nu Skin products for 16 years, since she was 59 and I was 32. But we had never imagined that we would have such incredible products. Thanks to Nu Skin, we can feel young and live a fulfilling life!

HISAYO AND MASA

Recently, I was exposed to ageLOC in a group sale my daughter organized for my friends. My daughter insisted I purchase product to encourage my friends to do the same. Finally, I caved in and purchased ageLOC Elements. I started using the set and fell in love with it. Today, I use ageLOC on a regular basis and enjoy the many compliments I get from people around me. I can't imagine my life without it.

MOR AND LILACH

I am an ageLOC Galvanic Spa fan. When I first heard that the ageLOC Transformation set had also been launched in China, I bought it immediately and use it regularly! After one month, I was surprised that the wrinkles around my eyes had faded and my eyes now look bigger than before—just like when I was young. My dark spots disappeared and my skin is more radiant. Now, every time I am out with my daughter, strangers think we are sisters instead of mother and daughter. ageLOC has restored my self-confidence and zest for life.

PEI YUN AND XIA

I have been looking for solutions for my skin. ageLOC not only helps me improve the color of my skin, but also restores its elasticity. When I go out with my daughter, people think we are sisters. I am thankful to my friend who introduced Nu Skin to me. Now I will introduce the Nu Skin products that help people appear more beautiful, healthier, and younger to my friends!

PING AND XIAO MENG

Since I started using ageLOC Galvanic Spa and ageLOC gels, everyone around me has said I look at least 10 years younger. My husband is also very happy. ageLOC Spa and ageLOC gels are the most effective products I have used in the past several years. My friends say my name should be Song Nian Qing ("help people become younger") instead of Song Qing Nian, because I have helped many friends look younger. This is my greatest achievement—more and more people are becoming younger, more beautiful, and more self-confident because of ageLOC and me.

QIN NIAN AND YAN NI

I think that the ageLOC products are fantastic, because not only do they make your skin look radiant and refined, but when used regularly, they help your skin look and feel years younger.

SHANIECE AND GABRIELE

My skin used to be dry and dull; I have not switched to any other brands after using Nu Skin products. It is not necessary to go to beauty salons anymore, once you have the ageLOC Galvanic Spa. After using ageLOC products, my skin is much better. When I am with my daughter, we look more like sisters! Becoming younger is not a dream anymore once you start using ageLOC!

XUE RONG AND ZHAN

Since I learned of Nu Skin 20 years ago, I have been a big fan of the products. I will continue to use ageLOC products for aging care and enjoy taking pictures like this 10 years, 20 years, and even 30 years from now.

YAYOI KIMURA

Every woman dreams of youthful, radiant, and healthy skin. You look in the mirror and dream of transforming at one stroke and getting radiant and youthful looking skin. I got this transformation with the help of ageLOC science. My friends tell me I look so much younger. In reality, there is no secret. Modern technologies and Nu Skin's cooperation with leading scientists have helped to provide these excellent results. That's why I have chosen ageLOC. I can keep my skin under control and am confident that I can keep my age a mystery.

TATIANA AND LYUBOV

These testimonials were provided by Nu Skin employees, distributors, customers, and guests.

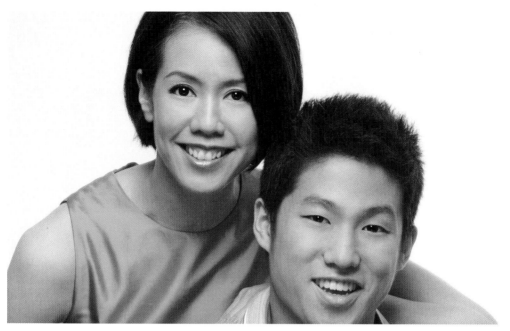

AMY AND GABRIEL, Singapore

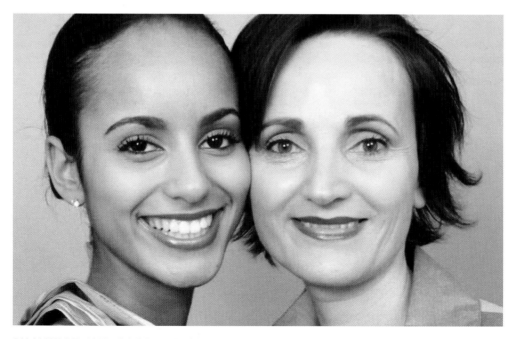

SHANIECE AND GABRIELE, Switzerland

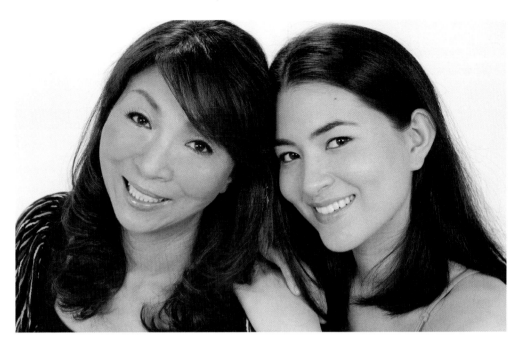

YAYOI AND ERIKA, Japan

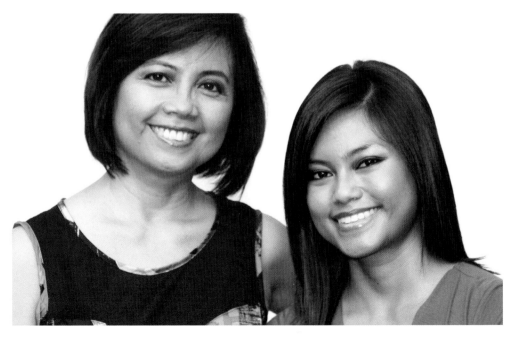

HAYDEE AND JANZ, United States

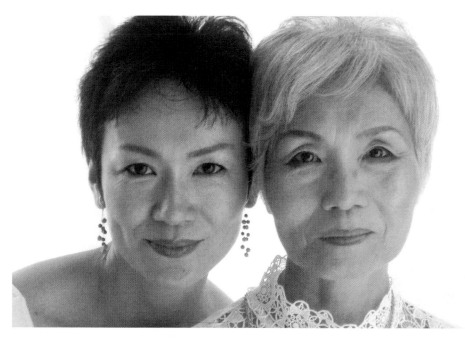

HISAYO AND MASA, Japan

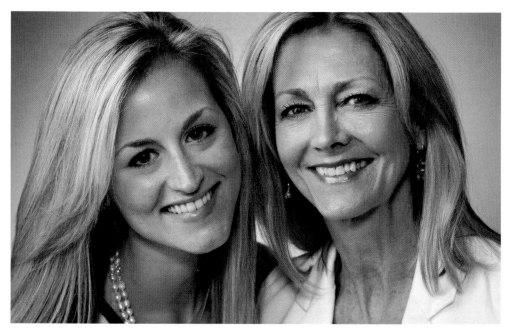

JOELLE AND CAROL, United States

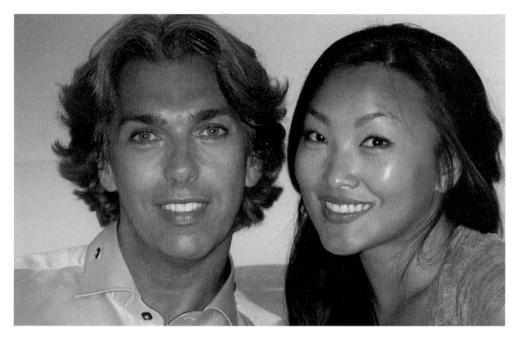

MASSIMILIANO AND ALEXIS, United States

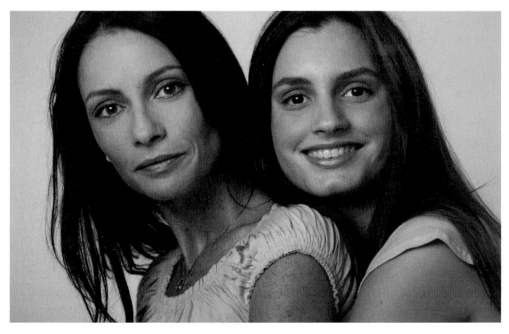

MOR AND LILACH, Israel

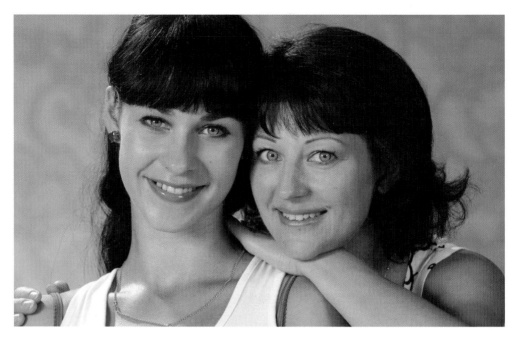

TATIANA AND LYUBOV, Russia

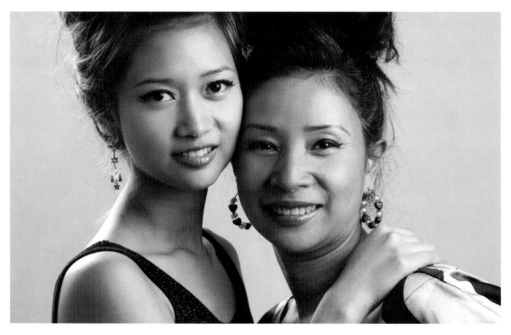

PIMPIRADA AND CHANUT, Thailand

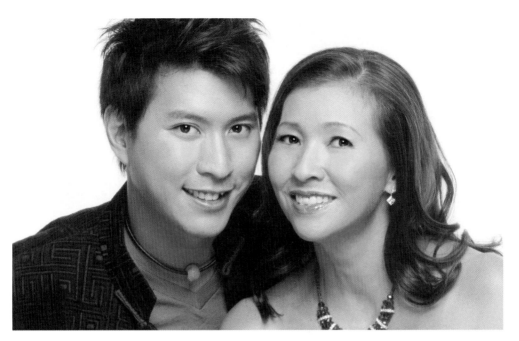

SAM AND PAULINE, Singapore

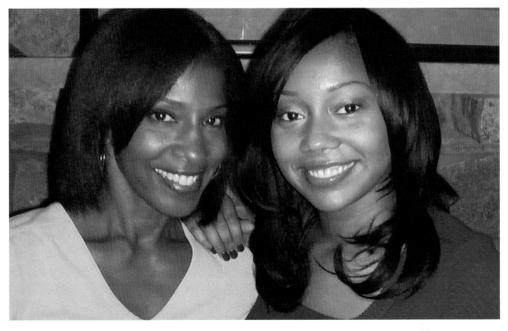

TERRI AND DOMINIQUE, United States

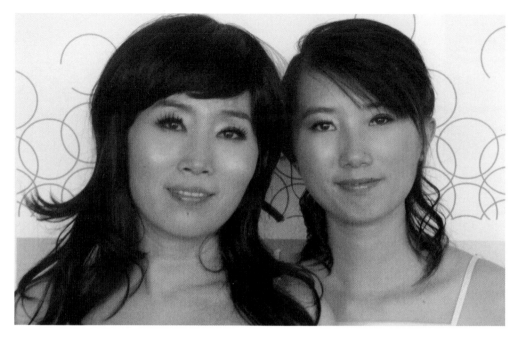

XUE RONG AND ZHAN, China

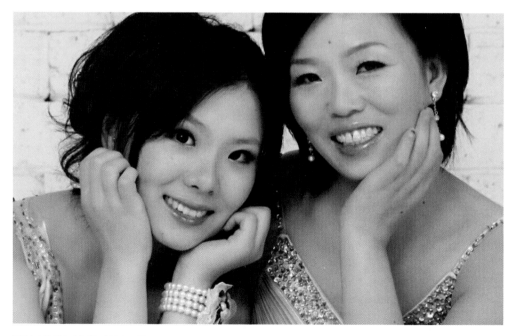

PEI YUN AND XIA, China

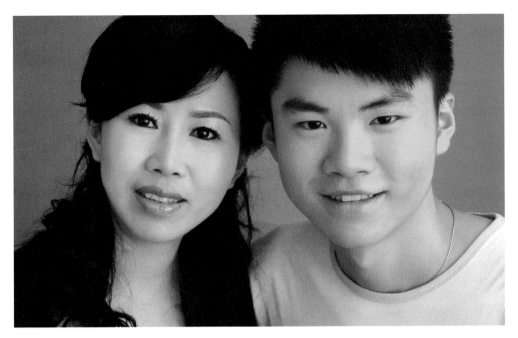

ZENG YU AND ZENG MING JIE, China

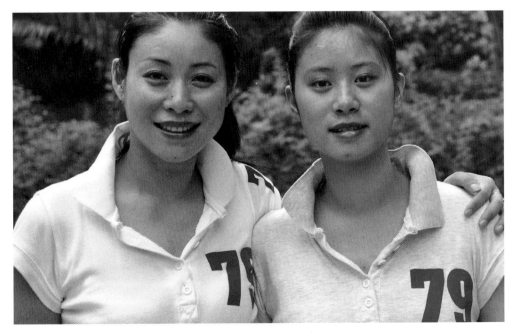

QIN NIAN AND YAN NI, China

NAME AND AGE	AGE DIFFERENCE
AMY **50** AND GABRIEL **18**	32
SHANIECE **17** AND GABRIELE **42**	25
YAYOI **54** AND ERIKA **20**	34
HAYDEE **58** AND JANZ **23**	35
HISAYO **48** AND MASA **75**	27
JOELLE **22** AND CAROL **59**	37
MASSIMILIANO **43** AND ALEXIS **28**	15
MOR **40** AND LILACH **21**	19
TATIANA **20** AND LYUBOV **40**	20
PIMPIRADA **20** AND CHANUT **44**	24
SAM **31** AND PAULINE **59**	28
TERRI **54** AND DOMINIQUE **25**	29
XUE RONG **44** AND ZHAN **17**	27
PEI YUN **19** AND XIA **41**	22
ZENG YU **41** AND ZENG MING JIE **19**	22
QIN NIAN **42** AND YAN NI **17**	25

AGELOC® YGC HEATMAP

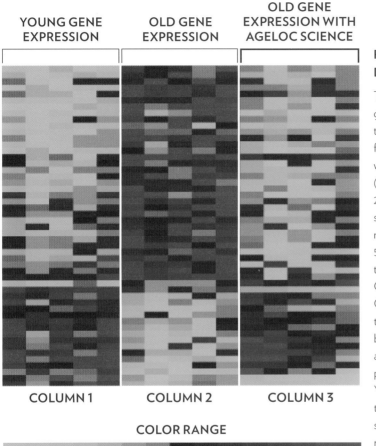

YOUNG GENE EXPRESSION

OLD GENE EXPRESSION

OLD GENE EXPRESSION WITH AGELOC SCIENCE

COLUMN 1

COLUMN 2

COLUMN 3

COLOR RANGE

LOW EXPRESSION

HIGH EXPRESSION

FIGURE DESCRIPTION

This heatmap illustrates gene expression of three groups of mice from a pre-clinical test with ageLOC. Young (column 1), old (column 2), and old with ageLOC science (column 3). Each row represents one of 52 genes comprising the mitochondrial Youth Gene Cluster (mtYGC). Columns 1 and 2 show that each of the 52 genes became more or less active during the aging process. In column 3, the YGC activity pattern of the old with ageLOC science group has been reset to a gene expression pattern more similar to the young group in column 1.

COLUMN 3 SHOWS HOW AGELOC SCIENCE **RESET** GENES TOWARD A MORE YOUTHFUL GENE EXPRESSION PATTERN.

Transcriptional Biomarkers of Mitochondrial Aging and Modulation by Cordyceps Sinensis Cs-4. Gordon Research Conference, Biology of Aging, Determinants of Health-Span: From Cells to Humans, August 22-27, 2010. Les Diablerets Conference Center, Les Diablerets, Switzerland.

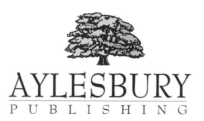